Prevention's

DIABETES

BREAKTHROUGHS

2008

Prevention's
DIABETES
BREAKTHROUGHS
2008

SMART SOLUTIONS FOR OPTIMAL
BLOOD SUGAR CONTROL

from the editors of **Prevention** magazine

RODALE

Printed in the United States of America
Rodale Inc. makes every effort to use acid-free ∞, recycled paper ♲.

Photo credits are on page 359.
Book design by Tara Long

ISBN-13: 978–1–59486–839–9
ISBN-10: 1–59486–839–5
2 4 6 8 10 9 7 5 3 1 hardcover

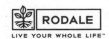

We inspire and enable people to improve their lives and the world around them
For more of our products visit **rodalestore.com** or call 800-848-4735

Contents

Part I

Take Control

Part II

Eat Right

Part III

Lose Weight

Part IV

Move It!

Part V

Stress Less

Part VI

Avoid Complications

Part VII

Diabetes Cookbook

Arm Yourself with Information

Seven percent of Americans—20.8 million of us—have diabetes. That's about the number of people who live in Pennsylvania and New Jersey *combined*.

Yet, because you've been diagnosed, you're ahead of many of them. Nearly one-third of the people with diabetes don't even know they have it. So they can't protect themselves against its deadly consequences.

And that's a scary thing. Diabetes is a condition that will slowly chip away at your health—at your life—unless you do something to fight back. That's where this book can help. It's filled with the latest information about diabetes, its challenges, and its complications. But most important, it's filled with the latest information to help you take back control of your health and your life.

In Part I, you'll learn how to "Take Control." It explains the basics of blood sugar and how it can affect your health when it's higher than it should be. It offers a wealth of information to help you protect your children from diabetes. (Type 2 diabetes used to be called adult-onset diabetes, and nearly all of its victims were older than 30. Now type 2 affects children as young as age 4, and the American Diabetes Association says this disease is approaching catastrophic proportions in teens.) You'll also learn about the mysterious condition called Syndrome X, of which diabetes is just the tip of the iceberg. And you'll find help in your search for "Doctor Right."

Part II will help you to "Eat Right." Discover a new approach to eating well with our Diabetes Diet. Get a glimpse inside the pantries of four top nutritionists as they share their real-world, study-backed tips. Learn what one item should be banned from your kitchen forever. And read about nine ways to chop, sauté, and stir your way to better health.

In Part III, you'll find our very best advice to "Lose Weight." The diabetes–weight loss connection is very strong. In fact, studies show an increase of less than half an inch in waist size could raise the risk of developing type 2 diabetes by a hefty 28 percent for women and 34 percent for men. If you struggle with your weight, this part of the book can help. Here you'll get slim, strong, and powerful with our 28-day program. You'll glean real-world tactics to survive the overeating season and discover how to survive the most common diet derailments.

Next, we hope that Part IV will inspire you to "Move It!" Burn calories, sculpt muscle, and shed fat with our workout plans. You'll feel slimmer the very first time you do our No-Sweat Slim Down.

Is stress a problem in your life? You're certainly not alone. Learn how to "Stress Less" in Part V. This is especially critical for people with diabetes because stress triggers hormones that raise blood sugar. The good news is that reducing chronic stress switches this process off. Find calm amid chaos and serenity amid stress with our expert tips.

Many complications are a terrible—and all too common—byproduct of diabetes. Learn how to "Avoid Complications" in Part VII. Here you'll find the latest breakthroughs on heart disease, depression, cancer, and more.

Finally, in Part VIII, the "Diabetes Cookbook," you'll find 100 delicious, nutritious diabetes-fighting meals and snacks. We hope that you—and your family—enjoy them all.

Hopefully, the information in this book will help you live your best life, despite diabetes. After all, information is power!

Part I

TAKE CONTROL

CHAPTER 1

HOW SWEET IT IS

The basics about your blood sugar

Stroll through the diet book section at Barnes & Noble and you'd think that blood sugar was the secret to ideal health and effortless weight loss: There's *The Sugar Solution, Get the Sugar Out,* and *Sugar Busters!* (to name a few). Which made us wonder: What is blood sugar anyway? And how important is it? To find out, we consulted the experts, pored over the latest research, and cut through the, um, BS.

FUEL FOR YOUR BODY

Let's say you're having a tuna sandwich for lunch. As soon as you finish eating, your digestive system starts breaking down the carbs—the lettuce, tomato, and whole wheat bread—into glucose. (In case you were dozing during Bio 101, glucose is a simple sugar found in plant and animal tissue.) Those glucose molecules race through your bloodstream, prompting insulin, a hormone made by your pancreas, to get in on the action. Think of insulin as your body's own personal UPS man (minus the foxy brown shorts): It scoops up the glucose in your blood and delivers it to sugar-hungry cells in your brain, muscles, and internal organs to use for energy. Insulin helps convert protein and fat into fuel, too, but glucose is "your body's most useful form of energy," says David L. Katz, MD, an associate professor at Yale School of Public Health. "It's really the only fuel that brain cells and red blood cells use."

To get enough glucose, your body depends on carbs like the US depends on foreign oil. That's why low-carb diets aren't a great idea for the long haul. "Although your body can process minimal energy from protein and fat, and your brain can use it in a real pinch—like to keep you alive in a famine—you don't want to count on them as your sole source," says Karen Chalmers, RD, a dietitian and advanced practice diabetes specialist at Harvard's Joslin Diabetes Center. "People who stay on low-carb diets long-term find their thinking becomes fuzzy" because their noggins don't have enough fuel.

So it's a good thing you're eating that tuna sandwich! Say you eat it at 1 p.m., and your insulin kicks into gear. In about 3 or 4 hours, the insulin has shuttled most of the glucose from your blood to your waiting cells. Your stomach starts to growl. If you don't eat anything by 5 or 6 p.m., you start to get really hungry—maybe even shaky, irritable, light-headed, or queasy. That's because your insulin has scraped up almost all the remaining glucose in your bloodstream, and your body's cells need more to keep chugging. Right now you probably have about 70 milligrams of sugar per deciliter of blood, versus a high of roughly 180 right after lunch (though numbers can vary widely depending on factors like your age, weight, overall health, and what you ate). Snack time!

You wander over to the office vending machine and buy a pack of Sno Balls. Hey, it happens. Minutes after you wolf them down, your blood sugar rockets up faster than it would take Borat to be ejected from high tea at Buckingham Palace. That sudden rush of glucose puts your pancreas into overdrive, inundating your body with insulin—which takes so much glucose out of your bloodstream at once that you crash, going from high to low blood sugar in as little as an hour. Result: You're crabby, jittery, starving, and craving more sweet treats to bring your energy—and your blood sugar—back up. "It's a vicious cycle," Dr. Katz says.

THE HEALTH CONNECTION

After a few years of eating a diet consistently high in Sno Balls and other refined carbs (think anything heavily processed or sugar laden that comes wrapped in plastic), your cells may start making like James Dean. They rebel against the blood sugar blitz by refusing to take any more glucose from your pushy insulin. That's a condition known as insulin resistance, also called prediabetes. So your pancreas, miffed, stops making enough insulin to get the job done.

But you're still downing Little Debbies, so the amount of glucose circulating in your blood begins to rise. The more pounds you pile on, the more your insulin starts to burn out and the higher your blood sugar gets—which can cause bigger problems than a bigger butt. We're talking the possibility of heart disease, stroke, and diabetes down the road. Reason: Excess blood sugar can increase the pressure your blood exerts on your organs, damaging them, says Walter Willett, MD, chair of the nutrition department at Harvard University School of Medicine and coauthor of *Eat, Drink, and Weigh Less.*

Exactly how much glucose is unhealthy? Scientists are trying to pin that down—it varies depending on family history and other risk factors (see "How Sweet Is Your Blood? Know Your BS," on page 6). But a 2006 study in the science journal the *Lancet* found that your risk for heart disease and stroke increases if your fasting blood sugar level (your blood sugar at its lowest, first thing in the morning before breakfast) is higher than 88 milligrams per deciliter (mg/dL). If it's between 100 and 125 mg/dL, you've got insulin resistance. It can make you feel cranky and

---

Butt Out

Who knew? Cigarettes are like skinny white Twix bars: Researchers aren't sure why, but smoking increases your blood sugar levels and decreases your body's ability to use insulin.

exhausted—and, if left untreated, can lead to type 2 diabetes, a serious condition where your body stops making enough insulin and which may require drugs for blood sugar management.

Okay, so high blood sugar is bad. But low blood sugar is no picnic either. If your glucose levels are consistently below 70 mg/dL, you have hypoglycemia, a condition that triggers feelings of nausea, dizziness, fatigue, and extreme hunger. Less than 1 percent of us have this problem, usually people who are genetically predisposed to it or on meds that can cause it. Though the long-term effects generally aren't as bad as for those with high blood sugar, ask your doc to test your glucose levels if you sus-

How Sweet Is Your Blood? Know Your BS

Check all the statements that are true for you.

_____ I am of African American, Native American, Asian, or Latin descent.

_____ My body looks more like an apple than a pear.

_____ My waist measures 35 inches or more.

_____ More than 10 percent of my daily calories (three or more servings) comes from simple sugars such as baked goods, candy, or sweets.

_____ I eat fewer than three servings of whole grains per day.

_____ My triglyceride levels are above 150.*

_____ My blood pressure is above 130/80.*

_____ My body mass index is over 25 (to calculate it, go to www.nhlbisupport.com/bmi).

_____ My mom, dad, or sibling has type 2 diabetes.

_____ My HDL (good cholesterol) is below 50, and my LDL (bad cholesterol) is above 100, or my total cholesterol is above 200.*

_____ I eat less than 24 grams of fiber per day.

_____ I smoke.

pect you have either condition. She may recommend drugs or an eating regimen to keep you feeling steadier.

SUGAR BUSTING

Which brings us to our main point: When it comes to staying healthy, getting blood sugar on your side is all about keep-ing it even-steven. That way it's available for the cells that need it but not taxing the rest of your body, and you don't have those panicky bring-on-the-doughnuts-now moments. A big part of that is eating the right foods at the right times.

Ideally, according to the National Heart, Lung, and Blood Institute, each meal will consist of 50 to 60 percent

0–4 TRUE: *Sugar star.* You can't choose your family or your ethnicity, both of which can predispose you to high blood sugar levels (though researchers aren't sure why). But you're doing a great job on the factors you can control. Sweet!

5–8 TRUE: *Sugar spiker.* You're chugging down the blood-sugar highway to the danger zone. Chronic high blood glucose and sluggish or erratic insulin make it harder for you to lose weight and may increase your risk for heart disease. That's why elevated triglyceride, cholesterol, or blood pressure levels should be as much of a wake-up call as a thickening waist or high BMI. Watch what you're eating to get yourself back on track and make sure your doc is monitoring your heart health.

9–12 TRUE: *Sugar-holic.* You're knee-deep in the vicious cycle of eating bad carbs, crashing, and eating some more. You're gaining weight (yet you never feel full), and your health is suffering. It's time to take charge of your eating habits and ask your doctor for a fasting glucose test. (Your fasting glucose levels, which are measured after 8 to 10 hours of not eating, are what doctors use to determine whether your blood sugar is too low or too high.)

---

*Your doctor should have these numbers on record if you don't know them offhand. Call her and ask.

What the Heck Is the Glycemic Index?

Many of the same fad diets that tell you to drop carbs like a bad habit also preach the glycemic index (GI), a system that assigns food a number per 50-gram serving based on how quickly you digest its carbohydrate content. For example, 50 grams of straight sugar has a GI of 100; 50 grams of apple has a GI of 55. The higher the GI number, the faster your blood sugar spikes and falls when you eat that food. (For a list of GI values, go to www.glycemicindex.com.)

Problem is, many people interpret the GI numbers incorrectly. "I'm not a fan of how the index gets used," says David L. Katz, MD. "Carrots have a high GI [131]. But you find me the person who is overweight because she ate carrots, and I'll quit my job and become a hula dancer." Don't feel compelled to check GI numbers before every bite, Dr. Katz says. "If you stick to whole foods [grains, nuts, seeds, fruits, vegetables, and lean meats] that are still close to their state in nature, the glycemic load of your diet will be low without you having to worry about it."

high-fiber carbs (such as fruits, veggies, and whole grains), approximately 15 percent protein (such as lean meats and fish), and 25 to 35 percent healthy fat (such as olive oil and nuts). You digest high-fiber carbs more slowly than refined ones, so your glucose levels will rise at a steady, leisurely pace and won't come careening down; they'll lower slowly over the course of 2 to 3 hours. Which is about how often you should eat—every 3 of your waking hours—to keep your blood sugar at an optimal level. Sounds like you'll be shoveling in more than Takeru Kobayashi at a Nathan's hot dog–eating contest, but you won't: If you sleep 8 hours a night, you've got 16 hours in the day, so you should eat about five times. Eat a small breakfast, lunch, and dinner and two snacks, and you're there.

GET MOVING

Working out also helps keep you level. "Exercising lowers your blood sugar because your muscles burn glucose when you move," Dr. Willett explains. "It also reduces insulin resistance almost immediately." In fact, in a study in the journal *Metabolism*, 12 weeks of aerobic training improved insulin sensitivity by 23 percent in overweight teenage girls. And that was before they even started losing weight.

Here's some diabetes-friendly exercise advice from the American Diabetes Association.

• Before you start an exercise program, talk to your health care team about what activities will be safe for you.
• Start slowly. Think about what activities are realistic for you.
• Check your blood glucose before and after exercising to learn how your blood glucose respond to exercise. Everyone's blood glucose responds differently to physical activity.
• Be cautious. If your blood glucose is high before you exercise (above 300), exercise can make it go even higher. (If you have type 1 diabetes, your fasting glucose level is above 250, and you have ketones in your urine, it's best to avoid exercise entirely.)
• Learn how to avoid low blood glucose, which can occur during or long after exercise.
• If you notice low blood glucose is interfering with your exercise, it may help to eat a snack before you exercise or adjust your medication. Consult with your health care team to find out what's best for you. For example, they might suggest you grab a healthy-carb snack such as a slice of whole grain bread or a piece of fruit about 90 minutes before you lace up your sneakers, since the immediate drop in blood sugar you experience during exercise can cause you to crash mid-run or be ravenous afterward. Also, having the right kind of fuel in your tank will help you work out better: In a recent study in the *International Journal of Sport Nutrition and Exercise Metabolism*, runners who breakfasted on All-Bran cereal and fruit ran 7 minutes longer than those who started the day with white toast, jam, and cornflakes.
• Drink plenty of water before, during, and after exercising.
• Wear a medical identification bracelet or necklace or a medical ID tag in case of emergency.
• Keep track of your progress to motivate yourself and help you meet your goals.

Chapter 2

AN EPIDEMIC ON THE MARCH

Here's everything you need to assess your diabetes risk—and safeguard yourself and your kids

It was early in the winter of 2004 when Jerry Silva first noticed things weren't right. Only 44 at the time, he'd drive home from his Boston-based research firm exhausted after a day of desk-jockey research analysis. He barely had the energy to greet his wife and daughter before collapsing on the couch for a predinner nap.

The weekends passed by in a blur. Often, Silva recalls, his fatigue was so overwhelming that he doubled up on naps, dozing for an hour or more in the midmorning and another couple of hours in the late afternoon. Yet he still felt tired all the time. He also felt dehydrated. But most of all, he felt out of shape—abysmally so.

During Silva's high school years in Indiana, the 6-foot-1 athlete had played football and worked out regularly, engaging in physical activities that ensured his big-boned body didn't go soft. Over the course of several decades—with marriage, the birth of his daughter, and the stresses of a cognitively challenging but physically undemanding occupation—Silva's weight gradually climbed to 273 pounds. It's a pattern familiar to legions of successful guys caught in the time crunches of middle age, when life on the go has little to do with actual movement.

Finally, Silva's wife advised him to see a doctor. Like all too many men (less than a third receive regular doctor exams), Silva hadn't undergone a physical in about 3 years. One test his doctor ran was a fasting blood glucose test (FBG), a measure of blood sugar levels after an overnight fast. In healthy people, the normal range is between 70 and 100 milligrams per deciliter (mg/dL). Silva scored 311—well above the 126 cutoff the American Diabetes Association (ADA) sets to diagnose type 2 diabetes.

"Until I had the test," says Silva, "I had no clue whatsoever. I had always felt that I was immortal. The moment I heard 'diabetes,' I lost my sense of immortality." Left untreated, diabetes can lead to a host of horrific complications—blindness, stroke, heart disease, amputations, erectile dysfunction in men—and eventually death.

Silva is one of an estimated 20.8 million Americans suffering from diabetes, about a third of whom haven't been diagnosed and receive no treatment, according to the National Institute of Diabetes and Digestive and Kidney Diseases. Another 54 million Americans have prediabetes, a condition with elevated blood sugar levels that raises the risk of developing type 2 diabetes. (Type 1 diabetes, despite its "primary" name, is far less common and accounts for approximately 5 to 10 percent of those who have diabetes. It's an autoimmune disease that is usually diagnosed in childhood.)

"Type 2 diabetes and the conditions that precede it, including obesity and prediabetes, represent the greatest epidemic we are facing in the 21st century," says David M. Nathan, MD, professor of medicine at Harvard and director of the Diabetes Center at Massachusetts General Hospital. Unlike a generation ago, type 2 diabetes isn't just stalking overweight thirty-somethings. Type 2 diabetes used to be called adult-onset diabetes, and nearly all of its victims were older than 30. Now type 2 affects children as young as 4, and the ADA says it is approaching catastrophic proportions in teenagers. Because of rising obesity and lack of exercise, the

The Essential Building Blocks

Choose the following smart food options for diabetes prevention.

Fish is a great source of unsaturated fats. Swedish researchers found that children who ate the most unsaturated fat—namely, the omega-3s found in fatty fish such as salmon, halibut, and tuna, as well as shrimp—were the least likely to be overweight, even though they were consuming more overall fat than their larger peers.

Vegetables like broccoli, celery, peppers, and tomatoes are essential for defeating diabetes, according to a study in the *American Journal of Epidemiology*, but only 27 percent of adults eat the recommended $2^1/_2$ cups of vegetables a day, according to the Centers for Disease Control and Prevention (CDC).

Whole grains are associated with decreased fasting blood sugar levels, according to a study in the *American Journal of Clinical Nutrition*. Refined grains, which have been stripped of the bran and germ and therefore have less fiber, are associated with increases in blood sugar.

Nuts regulate body weight and counteract cardiovascular and metabolic risk factors. A study published in the *Journal of Nutrition* found that eating almonds after a high-carb meal prevents spikes in blood sugar.

Fruit consumption is linked with a decrease in diabetes risk, according to a study in the journal *Preventive Medicine*. But only 33 percent of Americans get the recommended 2 cups of fruit a day, according to the CDC.

Dark chocolate could lessen your risk of developing diabetes, according to Italian researchers who determined that the flavonoids in dark chocolate can improve insulin sensitivity.

Centers for Disease Control and Prevention (CDC) recently predicted that at least one in three American children born in the year 2000 will develop diabetes at some point in his or her lifetime.

"Our worst fears are being realized," says David S. Ludwig, MD, PhD, director of the Optimal Weight for Life Program at Children's Hospital Boston. "People who were diagnosed as teenagers, who have had diabetes for 10 years and are now in their twenties, are developing life-threatening problems. And they're dying at a higher-than-expected rate."

But there are successful treatments, especially if they begin in the prediabetes stage. While the exact causes of type 2 diabetes are unknown, family history of the disease is a strong predictor. The essential first step is that adults learn to recognize the risk factors so that they can be tested and start treatment. If a father or mother is at risk, chances are the kids are, too. Diabetes is a family disease with family solutions. For those vested with reversing the diabetes epidemic, parents' abilities to teach their children is crucial: Family-oriented lifestyle changes may well offer the best chance for current sufferers to turn their lives around and for future generations to avoid the problem altogether.

CRACKING THE INSULIN ENIGMA

The first domino in the chain reaction that leads to prediabetes and eventually the full-blown disease is a phenomenon called insulin resistance. Put simply, body cells stop responding well to normal amounts of insulin, the hormone that allows glucose to pass from the bloodstream into the cells, where it is used for energy. Insulin is the physiological key that opens the locks lining the outside of cell membranes, allowing glucose inside. Though the exact mechanisms that cause type 2 are unclear, the insulin "key" itself appears unchanged. The "locks" on the cell membranes change or become blocked somehow, and they simply don't open when insulin comes calling. The net result is that glucose, like so much unloadable freight, piles up to toxic levels in the blood.

Put your finger into a bowl of table sugar and you'll find the little crystals can be quite sticky. "Glycation" is a fancy name for a similar stickiness that happens with glucose molecules in your bloodstream. Unable to enter the body's cells, they instead glom on to proteins in everything from red blood cells to blood vessel walls to nerves. Though some degree of glycation is natural, the higher the glucose levels in your bloodstream, the more danger you face. When glucose levels reach above 120 mg/dL, serious damage escalates, and a kind of sugar corrosion starts to interfere with virtually every major system in the body.

Researchers studying insulin resistance are struggling to find answers. Alan Sinaiko, MD, professor of pediatrics at the University of Minnesota Medical School in Minneapolis and a leader in insulin-resistance research, has studied children since 1996 to see if early changes in insulin sensitivity might predict diabetes in their future. (Insulin sensitivity is on the opposite end of the spectrum from insulin resistance and refers to cells that become adept at extracting nutrients and sugars from the bloodstream.) "It's true that the chance of seeing insulin resistance does go way up as kids approach obesity," he says. "But we found that thin kids can be insulin resistant, too, and that fat kids don't always have it. No one knows why insulin resistance develops." While excess body fat is considered the main

trigger, other suspected factors include genetics, environmental factors, and adipokines, highly inflammatory hormone-like substances produced by fat cells that some researchers believe are biochemical culprits for type 2, the way certain kinds of cholesterol are for heart disease. In 15 percent of type 2 diabetes cases, the cause is not traced to increased weight gain.

To check for impaired glucose processing, doctors use a range of tests, all of which measure blood sugar levels. Although most people don't know their numbers, chances are they have been tested. "Doctors usually throw in a glucose test anytime you go in for a physical or have blood drawn," says David M. Klurfeld, PhD, national program leader for human nutrition at the USDA. "But most will tell you the results only if they're abnormal." If, on the other hand, you haven't had your cholesterol measured or seen a doctor in several years, you should get checked out, especially if any of the following risk factors apply to you.

Obesity: The more fat you have, the more resistant your cells become to insulin. A body mass index (BMI) of 30 or higher more than doubles your risk for type 2.

Inactivity: A lack of exercise worsens insulin sensitivity.

Ethnicity: African Americans, Native Americans, and Latinos are almost twice as likely as Caucasians to develop the disease.

Depression: People who are depressed are more likely to get type 2 diabetes.

Family history: An estimated 45 to 80 percent of people with type 2 have at least one parent with the disease, and 74 to 100 percent have a first- or second-degree relative with the disease.

There's another reason to be aggressive about testing: A parent with elevated blood sugar levels is a red flag for doctors to test a child who might not ordinarily be examined. Most government agencies agree that widespread glucose testing in kids is not, at this point, warranted. "Screening all children for type 2 diabetes wouldn't be cost-effective," says Dr. Ludwig, "but I certainly advocate testing children who are at risk." This includes children 10 and older who are inactive, are significantly overweight, and have a strong family history of the disease. Some doctors also feel that testing spurs action. "People are much more frightened of diabetes than they are of obe-

sity," says Laura Svetkey, MD, director of clinical research at Duke University Medical Center. "If you do a blood test that shows the child has insulin resistance and explain what that means—that the child is prediabetic and can prevent diabetes through exercise and diet—you may be more likely to get everyone's attention."

Not long after his own diagnosis, Silva learned just what effect diabetes was having on his body. During a follow-up eye exam, ophthalmologist Deborah Eappen, MD, discovered minor damage to his retinas—another insidious side effect of blood sugar gone wild. Armed with the prescription drug Glyburide to help boost his insulin levels, Silva resolved to do everything he could to lose weight and get into shape. His first stop was Harvard Vanguard Medical Associates, where he met with a nutritionist. She advised him to commit to a lifestyle based on moderation in both nutrition and activity. He switched from regular soda to diet soda, knocked out fast food, and substituted complex carbs for simple carbs. To add some fun to his recommended exercise regimen of running for 30 minutes to an hour every day, he bought a treadmill and a flat-screen

Sugar Power

Our bodies burn an ever-shifting mix of carbs and fats for fuel. While the fat stores of even a 150-pound übermensch probably aren't in danger of depletion, carbohydrate stores fluctuate during exercise. The digestive system breaks down carbs into glucose, which enters the bloodstream. The process follows a general, if inexact, sequence.

Step 1

After several milliseconds of effort, muscle glycogen (the storage form of glucose) is broken down into glucose and burned during light exercise to fuel muscle contractions.

Step 2

As muscle glycogen stores gradually become depleted, muscle cells extract circulating glucose from the bloodstream to continue fueling contractions.

Step 3

As blood glucose levels dip, the liver receives a signal to start breaking down its glycogen stores and release glucose back into the bloodstream, where working muscle cells quickly snarf it up.

Step 4

Though fats are also being used as fuel, after half an hour or so, the percentage of fat burning increases, helping spare glycogen. Assuming there is no supplemental carb intake or continued intense exercise, blood sugar drops and glycogen stores eventually come close to depletion. The net result is fatigue and lack of coordination, what marathoners describe as "hitting the wall." Your body responds by inactivating muscle enzymes and even cannibalizing muscle in order to produce more glucose.

HDTV. He spent the next NFL season on his feet, running during the first half of football games, which he once used as a backdrop for napping. Within weeks, the combination of eating less and moving more resulted in noticeable changes in how he felt. After 2 months, he dropped 20 pounds, and his doctor took him off his insulin medication entirely.

THE MEDICINE-FREE CURE

As Silva's example illustrates, adopting a healthier lifestyle isn't just good medicine for type 2 diabetes, it's arguably the best medicine. The Diabetes Prevention Program (DPP), a landmark clinical trial, showed that even people at the highest risk can avoid disability or death, provided they are willing to make and maintain significant changes to their lifestyles.

The DPP study divided 3,234 volunteers with prediabetes into one of three groups. One-third received intensive lifestyle coaching designed to help them lose 7 percent of their body weight; they were told to eat less fat and fewer calories and add 150 minutes of moderate physical activity a week—for example, walking for 30 minutes 5 days a week. Another third received the powerful drug metformin, which slows the body's internal production of glucose, helping to lower blood sugar levels. The final third received placebo pills.

To the surprise of some, the lifestyle changes actually proved twice as effective as medication, and applying those changes to a family setting provides clear incentives for parents.

This is a good wake-up call for parents to be better role models for their kids, says James O. Hill, PhD, director of the Center for Human Nutrition at the University of Colorado Health Sciences Center. "In terms of healthy diet and physical activity, we know that whether the parents practice these habits is one of the best indicators of whether the kids will," he says.

Frequency of exercise is also important, because researchers have learned in recent years that any increase in physical activity will increase insulin sensitivity. "If you don't exercise again fairly soon, the sensitivity disappears over 1 or 2 days," says Dr. Nathan. "That's why we recommend that people exercise—for example, brisk walking or swimming

Sugar Tests

Ask your doctor for the following tests to determine how well your body uses blood sugar.

Fasting Blood Glucose Test

The FBG measures your blood glucose levels after 6 hours without food or liquids other than water.

Here are what the results mean.

Normal: less than 100 mg/dL

Impaired: (prediabetes): 100 to 125 mg/dL

Diabetes: 126 mg/dL or higher (cutoff lowered from 140 mg/dL in 1997 by the American Diabetes Association, or ADA)

Oral Glucose Tolerance Test

For the OGTT, following an overnight fast, you drink a sugary solution containing 75 grams of glucose, then have your blood levels measured over the next several hours.

Here are what the results mean.

Normal: blood sugar level less than 140 mg/dL within 2 hours

---

for 30 to 40 minutes—at least every other day, if not every day."

The Boukai family is living proof of just how effective lifestyle changes can be. In a follow-up study to see how to translate the DPP model into the real world, a team led by Ronald Ackermann, MD, of the Indiana University School of Medicine's Diabetes Prevention and Control Center, recruited volunteers from two YMCAs in Indianapolis. Gadi Boukai, 46, had moved from Israel to Indianapolis 7 years earlier, and the combination of less walking and more

Impaired: (prediabetes): blood sugar level between 140 and 199 mg/dL after 2 hours

Diabetes: blood sugar above 200 mg/dL after 2 hours

Glycated (or Glycosolated) Hemoglobin Test

Though generally not used to diagnose diabetes, the HbA1c, a test of how much glucose is bound to hemoglobin in your blood, helps doctors assess the effectiveness of your treatment plan. The more glycated your hemoglobin is (i.e., gummed up with sugar), the higher your average blood sugar has been over the past few months. In healthy individuals, this is generally 4 to 6 percent. In people with poorly controlled diabetes, it's 7 percent or higher. The ADA recommends treatment to keep this under 7 percent, which some doctors believe is too high.

A1C %	MEAN BLOOD SUGAR (MG/DL)
6	135
7	170
8	205
9	240
10	275
11	310
12	345

fast food made him put more than 20 pounds onto his 6-foot frame. His 44-year-old wife, Michele, gained significant weight after her children were born.

After testing, Gadi met the diagnostic criteria for entering the study. He weighed 216 pounds, his BMI was 29, and his fasting glucose was 107. Michele, at 5 feet 3 inches and 150 pounds, with a BMI of 27, didn't meet the necessary cutoffs, but she was encouraged to attend. And although the study was not designed to allow the kids to participate, the program's familial trickle-down effects also helped the Boukais' two "pleasantly plump" teenagers. Once a week for 16 weeks, the Boukais received cognitive-skills training in a host of areas, from grocery shopping for healthier choices to cooking tasty but lower-calorie meals to incorporating more exercise into daily life.

The details proved not just helpful but life changing for the Boukais. Gadi learned how to make better sense of product labels, and he discovered just how many calories his "healthy McDonald's choice," a fish sandwich, actually contained. On the physical-activity front, the parents learned to make a habit of new fitness routines; they joined a fitness center, where they now swim and play racquetball a few times a week. Gadi saw the powerful transformation in his kids firsthand during a Labor Day picnic. It was 6 months into the program, and Gadi and Michele found themselves tempted. "I was thinking, 'What the hell? It's just 1 day,'" recalls Gadi. "I could have consumed 3,000 to 4,000 calories easily. But then our kids came forward and said, 'Mom, Dad, do you really want to binge?' Michele and I decided the answer was no, and the four of us went for a walk instead."

THE LOW-CARB CONTROVERSY

The ADA has traditionally recommended a diet low in fat and rich in carbs such as grains, beans, and starchy vegetables. But many doctors are convinced that this simply isn't logical, because eating carbs—which quickly break down to glucose during digestion—impacts blood sugar levels more than protein, fat, or fiber does.

"When I first started looking at diabetes," says Eric C. Westman, MD, associate professor of medicine at Duke University and director of the Lifestyle Medical Clinic, "it made sense to me that you can positively influence the disease by reducing the carbohydrates." Supporters of the ADA disagree.

"The potential exists that the low-carbohydrate approach over years or decades could be harmful," says John Buse, MD, PhD, president-elect of the ADA. "The appropriate study has not been done, so discounting what has been demonstrated as safe and effective as inferior is foolish."

Dr. Westman concedes that studies to date on low-carb diets have involved much smaller numbers of patients and lack the statistical punch of the DPP, but the results are promising. The National Institutes of Health is currently funding a 5-year study comparing low-carb and low-fat diets in obese people.

Consider the case of 46-year-old Jeff Gerber, a bariatrician (a medical doctor who specializes in treating the overweight and obese) and family-practice physician in Denver. One of his first success-story patients was himself. "When I was 39," says the 5-foot-10 practitioner, "my weight had crept up from the 138 pounds I had weighed when running half-marathons a decade earlier to 205 pounds." The time-crunched father of three soon received more bad news: Several tests he ran on his blood sugar levels, though not yet placing him in the diabetic category, revealed he was well on his way. He decided to try the Atkins diet, slashing his carb intake while allowing himself as much protein and "healthy fats" as he wanted. Worried the latter might increase cardiovascular risk factors like cholesterol, he monitored his lipid profile religiously—and was surprised to see it actually got better, not worse. In fact, a recent Harvard School of Public Health study found that diets low in carbohydrates and high in protein and healthy fats actually reduce the risk of heart disease. Within a year, Dr. Gerber's

Sugary Statistics

No doubt about it, we're all too sweet on the sweet stuff.

26 pounds: amount of candy the average American ate in 2005

1.8 billion: number of candy canes eaten during the 6 weeks prior to December 25; laid end to end, would wrap around the earth nearly 10 times

73: percentage of teachers who use candy to reward students

235: number of calories, along with 6 grams of saturated fat, in 1.5 ounces of milk chocolate

2,404,237,000: pounds of sugar the US confectionery industry went through in 2005

450: number of varieties of soda sold in the United States weight dropped significantly—to a svelte 165 pounds. He was so inspired by his results that he now recommends a carb-restricted approach to his patients as well.

Devotees of both the low-carbohydrate and low-fat extremes duke it out in the literature with a fervor bordering on evangelism. Moderates in the debate suspect there is no one-size-fits-all answer here and that due to the differences in our genes, our metabolisms, and our culturally ingrained food preferences, what works to foster sustainable weight loss in one person might prove impossible for another to adhere to.

"I'd be willing to bet that over the next decade," says Dr. Klurfeld of the USDA, "we'll find 10 or 20 categories of gene clusters that will allow for individual nutritional and activity prescriptions." Person A, for instance, might do best by mixing a low-carb diet with a regimen of strength-training. Person B, on the other hand, should eat higher carbs and walk 2 miles a day.

But it matters less what you do than that you begin to take action. Just as Dr.

Gerber saw his condition improve with weight loss, so did the Boukai family. Gadi downsized from 216 pounds to 184, and his once high fasting glucose has normalized. Michele went from 150 pounds to 112. As for the kids, Gadi says one of his most rewarding moments was when his son asked him to run a 5K race with him at his school.

"My son easily beat me, of course," he says, "but I was so proud that we could do the run together."

After a year of working hard to get his diabetes under control, Jerry Silva shed 33 deadly pounds and lowered his A1c, a measure of the average amount of glucose in his blood over the past few months, from 10.3 to 6.5.

Today, instead of sedentary family activities such as watching movies, Silva and his family are doing active things, such as walking to a local park and flying kites, something his daughter loves. "At age 9," he says with obvious pride, "she can tell you which foods are carbs, fats, and protein." These are life lessons that are saving Silva—and guiding his loves ones.

CHAPTER 3

THE MYSTERY OF SYNDROME X

Some doctors say Syndrome X isn't a
disease at all. Others say more than
75 million Americans already have it.
But the medical community agrees on two
points: It will kill you, and the only person
who can cure it is you

At 4:30 in the dead calm of an unforgiving Missouri winter morning, Garry Tobin, MD, 47, shoulders his backpack, clips into his pedals, and powers his bike through the silent neighborhood of St. Louis' University City. No joyride, this. For Dr. Tobin, it's 40 minutes of self-prescribed cardio and musculoskeletal commuter medicine. With a family history of diabetes and obesity to contend with, he knows he needs to do all he can to prevent those small, seemingly harmless weight gains—a pound here, a pound there, the thickening inches of added girth that send men to the 34–36-waist, relaxed-fit jeans rack from the land of the 32 regulars. Or perhaps to the doctor. Or worse.

Dr. Tobin would know. He is the director of the Washington University Diabetes Center at Barnes-Jewish Hospital, where he fights weight every day—mostly other people's. He is well aware that carrying even a few extra pounds can lead to one of today's least known and yet most rampant diseases. So he rides, early and often, doing what he can in the predawn dark to move muscle and stack some odds in his favor.

"If diabetes is the tip of the iceberg," says Dr. Tobin, "then beneath the waterline is a constellation of related conditions that demand treatment."

He's talking about metabolic syndrome, or as some have dubbed it, Syndrome X. It's a disease marked by rising triglycerides in the blood, by elevated blood pressure, by increased insulin resistance—a laundry list of symptoms that seem to join forces to end people's lives. It has been lurking on the fringe of medicine for almost two decades now—a whole-body theory of health that draws a direct link between some of the most deadly diseases of our time—yet your doctor probably hasn't told you about it.

"Metabolic syndrome is the disease of the new millennium," says Steven Nissen, MD, chairman of the department of cardiovascular medicine at the Cleveland Clinic. "People with this cluster of symptoms have a disproportionate risk for heart disease," as well as diabetes and stroke.

It would be easy to dismiss metabolic syndrome as a new name for a bunch of old problems or, more cynically, a disease created to juice demand for new drugs. But the research is starting to pile up, and it suggests that a host of heart- and blood-related ailments are not only on the rise but also more closely connected than previously thought. It starts with symptoms that people tend to regard as the inevitable decay that comes with age: a few extra pounds, an increase in blood pressure. Then it slowly progresses until you suddenly have serious problems, such as insulin resistance, which can lead to diabetes, or increased triglyceride levels (fats in the blood), which can lead to a heart attack.

Today, according to scientists at the National Institutes of Health, some 75 million Americans have this serious condition. That's no small number. We're talking about the population of four Floridas—or 20 Oregons. Under different circumstances, we'd be looking at an epidemic of historic proportions. But since the symptoms are so closely related to existing diseases, doctors are arguing about how exactly to define metabolic syndrome and who exactly has it. As a result, not enough patients are being educated about the risks. Bureaucracy and politics may be to blame.

WHAT'S IN A NAME?

On one hand, the American Heart Association has urged doctors to recognize the disorder and take steps to help their patients control it. "Metabolic syndrome is the fastest-growing condition in the world," says John Foreyt, PhD, of Baylor College of Medicine, "and it would be unfortunate if politics were to get in the way of diagnosis." He's taking a not-so-subtle jab at opponents such as the American Diabetes Association (ADA), which says there isn't enough evidence to back up a diagnosis.

Some call it a turf war. "I believe the American Diabetes Association sees a strong overlap between metabolic syndrome and its two major themes: prediabetes and diabetes," says Scott Grundy, MD, PhD, director of the Center for Human Nutrition at the University of Texas Southwestern Medical Center.

"It's possible that the two organizations are competing for the same financial resources."

Richard Kahn, PhD, chief scientific and medical officer of the ADA, dismisses metabolic syndrome as nothing more than a new name for a bunch of existing ailments. "It's two words put together to make a term," he says. "There's no evidence that we've defined metabolic syndrome in any logical, evidence-based manner."

Grouping these risk factors together, Dr. Kahn argues, doesn't confer better treatment or longer life to those who are purportedly afflicted.

Even Gerald Reaven, MD, the Stanford scientist credited with discovering metabolic syndrome, who said that "half of all heart attacks are caused by Syndrome X," has changed his tune. He now calls the syndrome a ludicrous idea. Doctors don't need a catchall term like metabolic syndrome to protect patients' health, he says. They need to know whether a patient has high blood sugar.

"The diabetes community seems to think the only thing that's important is blood sugar. Frankly, I think that view is much too narrow," says Dr. Nissen. "This is a lot of misplaced energy, when what we really want to know is, what can we do for people who have these risk factors?" Get past the semantics, he says, "and there is a simple reality here: If you have at least three of these features, you're at greater risk for developing type 2 diabetes, coronary heart disease, heart attack, and stroke." Here are those risk factors.

- **Hypertension:** high blood pressure (130/85 millimeters of mercury—mm HG—or above)
- **Hyperglycemia:** fasting blood sugar equal to or more than 100 mg/dL or evidence of prediabetes
- **High triglycerides in the blood:** blood fats that promote plaque buildup in the arteries
- **Low levels of HDL** (good) cholesterol
- **Excess abdominal weight:** waistline greater than 40 inches for men; 35 for women

All the doctors agree that these symptoms tend to cluster, but some point to fat around the midsection as one of the most important factors. "Simply putting enough inches on your waist often leads to insulin resistance and thus will cause you to end up with metabolic syndrome," says James Kenney, PhD, nutrition research specialist at the Pritikin Longevity Center in Florida.

Most people think fat is simply ugly. Even doctors used to see it as nothing more than an inert storage depot. But the latest research suggests that it's actually dangerous.

Fat is an "incredibly active tissue," says Richard Weindruch, PhD, a professor of medicine at the University of Wisconsin–Madison Institute on Aging who studies the effects of calorie restriction on longevity. "It acts almost as another endocrine organ in the body, producing biologically active molecules that increase the risk for metabolic syndrome."

Among these biologically active molecules is one called adiponectin, which helps regulate insulin sensitivity, a key factor in metabolic syndrome and diabetes. Insulin, a hormone secreted by the pancreas, is what allows our bodies to process blood sugar, or glucose, for energy. Insulin is also responsible for sending excess glucose to the liver, where it's shelved as glycogen for later use.

Insulin sensitivity is the measure of how well your body uses glucose for energy. The higher your sensitivity, the more efficiently your body uses glucose and the lower your risk of diabetes. The problems start when people develop increased levels of visceral fat, the kind of fat that sits behind the abdominal muscles and surrounds your internal organs. As these fat levels go up, amounts of adiponectin decrease, and that can throw your insulin sensitivity out of whack, according to Dr. Weindruch. As a result, your blood sugar spikes and the pancreas responds by cranking out extra insulin, which can lead to type 2 diabetes.

Redefining fat as a dangerous affliction could have a major impact on our health system. Under current rules, the government won't pay for weight loss drugs, says Dr. Nissen, because it considers obesity a cosmetic problem. "People are developing drugs that they would like to use to treat metabolic syndrome," he explains, "but the FDA turns around and says, 'If you guys can agree on defining it, we'll let you develop drugs to treat it.'"

But agreement has been hard to come by, and, as a result, pharmaceutical companies have less incentive to address the problem directly, Dr. Nissen contends. "So if I can demonstrate that losing weight with a drug actually slows the progress of atherosclerosis,

that would be a very important development," he says.

Drug companies would certainly agree. Indeed, with 75 million potential patients, some pharma firms have decided it's worth taking the risk that the FDA will come around. In the meantime, there are plenty of other markets. Sanofi-aventis recently secured approval in Europe and Argentina for the first drug to treat metabolic syndrome: rimonabant, which is also known by its brand name, Acomplia, or simply as the "thin pill." The drug works by blocking receptors in the brain that have been shown to control appetite. Analysts are optimistic that the FDA will eventually approve the drug here. Sanofi is reviewing its safety testing in response to FDA concerns (including questions about psychological side effects).

How effective will rimonabant be in treating metabolic syndrome? Depends on whom you ask. Many of the doctors who don't think the syndrome is a legitimate condition write off the drug as a weight loss treatment and nothing more. But Dr. Nissen contends that rimonabant seems to have an effect on the fat cells themselves. He is conducting a study at the Cleveland Clinic to determine if the drug can slow the progression of coronary atherosclerosis, or plaque buildup in the heart. "If it works," says Dr. Nissen, "then who cares what you call the disease?"

FAT-FIGHTING 101: DIET

Even though metabolic syndrome may not show up on your doctor's radar until pharmaceutical companies start pitching a drug for it, there's a treatment available now: diet and exercise. "Medications don't solve the underlying problems," says Dr. Grundy. "This is a lifestyle issue, and increased physical activity and a healthier diet will treat all the risk factors at once."

According to the American Heart Association, in 2004, the latest year for which they have statistics, 79,400,000 Americans have one or more forms of cardiovascular disease. In 2004, it killed 871,500 (36.3 percent of all deaths). According to the American Diabetes Association, 20.8 Americans, or 7 percent of the population, have diabetes. While an estimated 14.6 million have been diagnosed, unfortunately, 6.2 million people (or nearly one-third) are unaware that they have the disease. Met-

abolic syndrome is what happens before these deadly diseases set in.

"The main driver of the syndrome is all of us getting heavier and heavier," says Dr. Foreyt.

While many factors can contribute to weight gain, the actual cause is simple: taking in more calories than you burn. We all have three "burns" that make up our metabolism, no matter how much we exercise.

Basal (resting) Metabolism: This is the largest burn rate—up to 80 percent of your daily calorie burn—and, surprisingly, it is the number of calories you burn doing nothing at all: lying in bed staring at the ceiling, or watching a PowerPoint presentation. It is fueled by the inner workings of your body—your heart beating, your lungs breathing, and even your cells dividing.

Exercise and Movement Metabolism: This includes both workouts at the gym and countless incidental movements throughout the day, such as turning the pages of this book. It accounts for 10 to 15 percent of your daily burn.

Digestive Metabolism: Also known as thermic effect of food (TEF), simply digesting food—turning carbs into sugar, and protein into amino acids—

typically burns 10 to 30 percent of your daily calories. Protein burns more calories during digestion—about 25 calories for every 100 consumed—while carbohydrates and fat burn about 10 to 15 calories for every 100 consumed.

When USDA scientists studied the eating habits of 8,837 adults, they found that on a typical day, overweight adults eat a mere 100 calories more than their normal-weight peers—the equivalent of having a cookie with your 3 p.m. coffee. But that cookie could be the problem. According to a National Center for Health Statistics study on dietary intake trends in the United States, people are consuming 60 grams more of carbohydrates every day than they did 20 years ago. Increased carbohydrate consumption could be the single biggest contributor to our ever-expanding waistlines, says Jeff Volek, PhD, nutrition and exercise researcher at the University of Connecticut at Storrs.

Scientists at the University of Florida recently determined that dieters who ate less than 100 grams of carbohydrates daily lost an average of 4 pounds more fat per month, compared with those whose carb intake was higher. This figure was based on a restricted-calorie diet, so for people on a standard regimen—say, 2,000 calories a day—175 grams would constitute a reduced-carb diet.

"Decreasing carbohydrate intake," says lead researcher James Krieger, "decreases the levels of insulin, a hormone that signals your body to store fat." For reference, one slice of whole grain bread has 12 grams of carbohydrates, and a cup of high-fiber vegetables—such as broccoli or green beans—has about 6 to 8 grams.

But as with most things concerning metabolic syndrome, the experts are divided when it comes to carbohydrates. Paul Jacques, DSc, of the Jean Mayer USDA Human Nutrition Research Center on Aging at Tufts University, points to a study in the journal *Diabetes Care*. "Those who ate the highest amounts of whole grains showed the lowest levels of metabolic syndrome," he says. Add to that the findings from a major clinical trial called the Diabetes Prevention Program (DPP), which showed that diabetes risk goes down when you exercise and eat a low-fat, high-carb diet, and you can see why there's no consensus.

Dr. Volek, a member of the low-carb crew, says a close look at the DPP study suggests that weight loss and exercise are the key factors in reducing diabetes risk, not carbs. "All the symptoms of metabolic syndrome respond to low-carbohydrate diets," says Dr. Volek, who coauthored a paper on the subject in the medical journal *Nutrition and Metabolism*. That doesn't mean you have to go to Atkins extremes, however.

"The typical American eats only one serving of whole grains each day, so there's room left for whole grains in the diet as long as it's within limits," says Dr. Volek.

But starchy foods—bread, pasta, rice—are a problem. "Starch turns into glucose the same way sugar does," says Keith Berkowitz, MD, founder of the Center for Balanced Health in New York City. "Focus on carbohydrates that are high in fiber and low in refined carbs, such as greens, fruits, and vegetables. These fiber-rich foods don't promote the insulin response that other carbohydrates do, because fiber isn't absorbed into the body, so you're satiating yourself without affecting your blood sugar."

A wonderful side effect is that when you approach food this way, the calories take care of themselves. "When people restrict carbohydrates in their diets, they usually don't replace those calories with fat or protein," says Dr. Volek. In a recent study he conducted, participants were asked simply to restrict carbohydrates; by doing so, they actually decreased their calorie intake by 800 calories a day.

FAT-FIGHTING 102: EXERCISE

The more scientists study the issue, the more indication there is that carbs wreak havoc on our bodies if we don't keep them in check. But diet isn't the only defense; exercise is extremely important, too. That's because carbs are stored in your muscles as glycogen, and when you're not expending a lot of energy, your glycogen tank fills up. The excess carbs not only elevate blood sugar but also head to your liver, where they're converted into triglycerides, which turn into visceral fat. This is one reason why hitting the gym is such a powerful tool in the fight against metabolic syndrome. In addition to the short-term benefit of burning up those excess carbs, you'll also build muscle, which will enlarge your storage capacity for carbs, says Dr. Volek.

And here's the beauty of it: When your

glycogen tank is low, your body's priority is to fill it again. This means that after intense exercise, your body has to burn fat (instead of carbs) for energy so that it can rebuild its glycogen stores. That's one of the main reasons your body burns fat at a higher rate after high-intensity exercise, compared with low-intensity exercise.

But on the reverse side, if your glycogen stores are full (from a lack of activity), your body assumes there are plenty of incoming carbohydrates available for energy, so it has no need to burn fat.

To really stoke your carb-burning furnace, hit the weights. The more muscle you work, the more calories you'll burn, says Christopher Scott, PhD, author of a study on the subject at the University of Southern Maine. You'll not only burn as many calories (or more) per minute as you would with intense aerobic exercise, but you'll also see more lasting benefits. In fact, a study from the Human Performance Laboratory at the University of Wisconsin–La Crosse showed that you can boost your metabolism for nearly 40 hours with only four sets each of three exercises.

Adding muscle is your best defense against dangerous midlife pounds. Studies show that people lose about 1 percent of their muscle mass per year, beginning at midlife. And a few extra pounds of fat around the middle can actually sabotage the muscle you've worked hard to build. A study published in the *Journal of Applied Physiology* showed that those biologically active molecules released from visceral fat can degrade muscle quality. That's why it's so crucial to target and destroy it. "This is dangerous fat," says Dr. Tobin, the commuting cyclist, "and when you lose it, you lose it from inside the organs, which will drastically improve your metabolic profile."

Dr. Tobin has the same 31-inch waist at age 47 that he had at 20, and he's still packing on muscle. In other words, he's moving in the right direction, every weekday morning, through the dark streets of St. Louis.

CHAPTER 4

SPECIAL REPORT: TYPE 1 DIABETES AND YOUR IMMUNE SYSTEM

Here's what you need to know to maximize your immunity and live well with type 1

Most people probably wouldn't think there's a connection between diabetes and the immune system. And for type 2 diabetes, they'd be right! However, the less common type 1 diabetes is intimately connected to the immune system.

When most people hear the word *diabetes,* they tend to think of type 2, the most common type among the 20.8 million Americans with diabetes. It results from insulin resistance, a condition in which the body can't properly use insulin, the hormone that "unlocks" the body's cells and allows glucose (blood sugar) to enter and fuel them.

However, of the total population with diabetes, about 5 to 10 percent have type 1. In this version, the body is unable to produce its own insulin because the beta cells in the pancreas—the only cells in the body that can make insulin—have been destroyed.

Until recently, type 1 diabetes was thought to affect primarily children and young adults (hence its alternative name, juvenile diabetes). But now more adults are being diagnosed with type 1. "You can see forms of it develop in people up to age 90," says Claresa Levetan, MD, clinical professor at the Lankenau Institute for Medical Research at Lankenau Hospital in Wynnewood, Pennsylvania.

Among the symptoms of type 1 diabetes are increased thirst and urination, weight loss despite increased appetite, nausea, vomiting, abdominal pain, fatigue, and absence of menstruation. Left untreated, type 1 diabetes can lead to serious complications such as heart disease, blindness, and nerve and kidney damage.

THE TYPE 1–IMMUNITY LINK

Unlike type 2 diabetes, which is a metabolic disorder, type 1 has a very strong link to the immune system. Specifically, the immune system is responsible for destroying the insulin-producing beta cells. In other words, type 1 diabetes is an autoimmune disease.

"An autoimmune disease occurs when the immune system makes a mistake and starts attacking the body's own cells and tissues," explains Alberto Pugliese, MD, research associate professor of medicine, microbiology, and immunology and head of the immunogenetics program at the Diabetes Research Institute at the University of Miami Miller School of Medicine. "Some people have multiple autoimmune diseases, while others have one disease that affects multiple organs.

"Type 1 diabetes is a classic example of an organ-specific autoimmune disease," Dr. Pugliese adds. "It affects only one organ—the pancreas. And even within that organ, it targets just the beta cells."

But what causes the immune system to run amok? According to Dr. Levetan, it's a combination of genetic predisposition and an environmental trigger. "If you have a genetic predisposition to type 1 diabetes, it means that there is a mistake in your immune mechanism," she explains. "So let's say that you get an illness such as the mumps. Your body will make antibodies to fight the mumps. After you've gotten over the illness, the antibodies will begin attacking the beta cells in the pancreas because of that mistake in the immune mechanism. Once you've lost 90 percent of your beta cells, you no longer have the ability to process glucose."

PROTECT YOURSELF

Doctors have come to view type 2 diabetes as a lifestyle disease, meaning that certain lifestyle choices—especially diet and exercise—can influence risk for better or worse. Not so with type 1 diabetes.

"We know that a person must have the genetic predisposition in addition to the environmental trigger, but we don't know what the trigger might be," Dr. Levetan says. "We've seen some associations with babies who were fed cow's milk in their first year and with people who have low levels of vitamin D. But for now, we can't do much to prevent type 1 diabetes."

One strategy that you may want to try: Battle vitamin D deficiency, which appears to contribute to autoimmune disorders such as type 1 diabetes. It's on the rise in the United States, at least partly due to our indoor, sunlight-deprived society.

"In a study of more than 10,000 children, researchers found that those who took a recommended dose of vitamin D during infancy were far less likely to develop type 1 diabetes than those who did not," says Rallie McAllister, MD, MPH, a board-certified family physician and author of *Healthy Lunchbox: The Working Mom's Guide to Keeping You and Your Kids Trim*. "Although some foods are fortified with vitamin D, the amounts are relatively low. It's probably best to take a supplement."

But how much to take is the subject of great debate. "According to the Institute of Medicine, kids under age 19 and adults under age 50 should get 200 IU of vitamin D a day, adults ages 51 to 70 should get 400 IU a day, and adults older than age 71 should get 600 IU a day," Dr. McAllister says. "Among nutrition experts, these recommended daily intakes are widely believed to be inadequate. Many experts recommend a daily intake of 1,000 IU for adults [over age 19]."

HEAL YOURSELF

People with type 1 diabetes need insulin to survive (which is why you may hear it described as insulin-dependent diabetes).

It's different from type 2 diabetes, in which the body makes insulin but the hormone isn't working as it should. If you have type 1, you should definitely work closely with your doctor to develop and fine-tune your treatment plan. The following measures may help balance your blood sugar and prevent diabetes complications down the road.

Be healthy. "The best things to complement the treatments that your doctor prescribes are the same things that anyone should do to maintain good health," says Luigi Meneghini, MD, associate professor of clinical medicine and director of the Eleanor and Joseph Kosow Diabetes Treatment Center at the Diabetes Research Institute at the University of Miami Miller School of Medicine. "Eat reasonably, exercise regularly, and maintain an ideal body weight."

Check and recheck. "It's critical for people with type 1 diabetes to monitor their blood sugar levels throughout the day," Dr. Levetan says. "Keep a journal of what foods you eat and how your blood sugar levels change to understand how your body responds to different foods. That way, you can tailor the insulin that you take to mimic what your own pancreas would do. Every 10 min-

utes, the pancreas releases a burst of insulin; within 1 minute of eating, it makes the perfect amount of insulin. You want to do as much as you can to follow that pattern."

Chill out. People with type 1 diabetes need to learn how stress affects their blood sugar. "During times of stress—both psychological and physiological, such as illness—your body releases stress hormones, which raise blood sugar levels," Dr. Meneghini explains. "So when you're under stress, there's a good chance that your blood sugar levels will rise. For some people, it can be as much as 200 to 300 mg/dL [milligrams per deciliter of blood]. It depends how sensitive you are to stress.

"Also, during times of stress, your body may not respond to insulin as it usually does," Dr. Meneghini adds. "So you need to check your blood sugar level more often, take insulin more frequently, and increase your dose if necessary. When the stress goes away, go back to what you were doing before."

Move it. Historically, studies have shown that people with type 1 diabetes live longer if they exercise regularly. More recently, the Finnish Diabetic Nephropathy Study found that women

(continued on page 38)

Future Type 1 Treatments

Researchers who study type 1 diabetes say the future looks bright. "I hope that we will have a cure for type 1 diabetes in our lifetime," says Alberto Pugliese, MD, research associate professor of medicine, microbiology, and immunology and head of the immunogenetics program at the Diabetes Research Institute at the University of Miami Miller School of Medicine. "For sure, we will have treatments and other measures that will have an even greater impact on the condition than the ones we already have." Here's just a sampling.

Better diagnostic measures: Researchers know that when immune cells attack beta cells, they're responding to specific molecules that beta cells make. "We call these target molecules," Dr. Pugliese says. "In many patients, one of the target molecules actually is insulin itself. This explains in part why beta cells are the only cells killed off. It's as though insulin is waving a flag and saying, 'Come shoot me.'

"Now that we know what some of these target molecules are, we know what the immune system goes after," Dr. Pugliese adds. "So we are learning how to identify people who are developing type 1 diabetes, before they even have symptoms, by measuring certain markers in their blood. These markers are the antibodies that are directed against the same target molecules that the lymphocytes go after. Sometimes these antibodies are present years before symptoms develop, when insulin production appears to be normal."

Improved treatments: As researchers are able to determine at an earlier stage who will develop type 1 diabetes, their next step is to find ways to disrupt and perhaps even halt the disease process. "One possibility is to put a person on immunosuppressive drugs," says Dr. Pugliese, who has participated in a number of clinical trials. "The problem with this treatment is that it may work for a time, but then the disease comes back. Also, the drugs suppress all of the immune cells, not just the small number causing trouble. The drugs can have a lot of unpleasant side effects, so they could not be taken indefinitely."

Current trials are exploring the use of immunosuppressive medications for a limited time and with an emphasis on immune regulation rather than immune suppression.

Another possibility is to treat people with one or more target molecules to help regulate the immune system and specifically control the "bad" immune cells that kill off beta cells. "In one double-blind, randomized study, the Diabetes Prevention Trial, we found a significant effect in people who had developed antibodies to insulin," Dr. Pugliese notes. "We're going to expand this study in the near future."

Ultimately, Dr. Pugliese says, the best approach may be a combined one. "We may treat people with one or more target molecules—insulin, for example—and also with immune-suppressing drugs for short periods. The goal is to get rid of the immune cells that destroy beta cells with drug therapy, while regulating the immune system with administration of the target molecules. Perhaps once the immune system stops destroying beta cells, we'll see regeneration or the formation of new beta cells."

Islet transplants: Islets are clusters of cells in the pancreas that consist of several types of cells, including the beta cells that produce insulin. In a study conducted by the National Institutes of Health, 60 percent of people with type 1 diabetes who underwent islet transplants didn't need daily insulin shots a year later. The downside is that transplant patients need to take powerful immune-suppressing drugs for life, which come with a host of nasty side effects. Also, islet transplants begin to lose functioning after a year. Further research may help troubleshoot and refine this experimental procedure.

with type 1 diabetes who did not exercise had worse blood sugar control than women who did. But you need to be smart about how you exercise—and definitely talk to your doctor before you start a fitness routine.

"People with type 1 diabetes need to be mindful of how exercise affects their blood sugar levels," Dr. Meneghini says. "The combination of exercise and high insulin levels tends to lower blood sugar much more than either exercise with basal insulin levels or no exercise. For example, let's say that you're planning to eat a meal containing 60 grams of carbohydrates, and your blood sugar level is 200. You calculate that you need to take eight units of insulin. If you're planning to exercise within a couple of hours of taking the insulin, you may need to reduce your dose.

"We give patients with type 1 diabetes some guidelines about how exercise affects blood sugar levels and some suggestions about how to alter their insulin dosing. But since everyone responds differently to exercise, the rest is trial and error," Dr. Meneghini adds. "For instance, one patient of mine—a high school basketball player—noticed that his blood sugar level would go low during practice, but it would go high during a game. The higher adrenaline levels during his games were pushing up his blood sugar level."

CHAPTER 5

THE SEARCH FOR DOCTOR RIGHT

Here's how to get the health care you deserve

Prisciliana Porras, 39, of Grapevine, Texas, was at risk of a serious health problem, and she didn't know it. Diagnosed at 21 with endometriosis, she'd had several surgeries and three children and had taken various hormone treatments. Yet until 3 years ago, when she wondered out loud at a checkup if she might be depressed, not one of her doctors had ever thought to ask about how she was coping, whether she felt anxious, or whether she was getting enough sleep—though her chronic, painful illness and subsequent surgeries put her at high risk of clinical depression. Thanks to antidepressants, Porras's fluctuating moods and anxiety have evened out, but she resents not getting treatment sooner. "I probably suffered with undiagnosed depression for 16 years, until it finally occurred to me to say, 'I think I need some help,'" she says.

Porras's case is a classic example of how great the divide can be between patients and doctors and how much can go wrong—even when patients are informed and assertive and doctors are skilled and caring, says Mack Lipkin Jr., MD, a professor of medicine at New York University School of Medicine.

It's a matter of hesitation on both sides. "Patients are afraid they won't be taken seriously, so they don't speak up," says Dr. Lipkin. And doctors are often muzzled by their own worries. "We're thinking, 'What if I make a mistake? What if I miss something? What if this takes forever?'"

The result is that the typical doctor-patient relationship is based on fractured communication—usually just frustrating, sometimes downright dangerous. In a study of more than 1,000 exchanges, published in the *Journal of the American Medical Association* in 1999, doctors failed to give patients enough information to make informed treatment choices in an astounding 91 percent of cases. The result can be harmful, even life threatening: Patients who don't get clear answers on why and how they should use prescribed medicines, for instance, are less likely to follow through on taking them.

But poor communication isn't the only thing eroding the bond between you and your doctor. The advent of managed care has resulted in less choice in whom you can see; it also means that your physician is probably taking on more patients than ever, might be running late, and may be holding shorter appointments. Evidence also suggests that doctors enjoy their jobs less than they ever did in the past, and patients may switch providers more than once. All of these factors could add up to substandard medical care, even from a perfectly qualified health care professional. But there are ways savvy patients can get more from their doctors—without shelling out one extra cent.

Here's a 10-point list of demands you have the right to make of your doctor, with suggestions for how to make them happen, followed by what she wishes she had the time (and the nerve) to say to you. In all, 18 ways to build the kind of health care connection that will help keep you healthier and both of you happier.

DOCTOR, PLEASE . . .

1. Don't make me wait. Nearly half of all Americans say they spend too much time cooling their heels in their doctor's waiting room, making it the most common health care complaint, according to a 2003 *Wall Street Journal* Online/Harris Interactive Health-Care Poll. And while waiting never hurt anyone (okay, maybe your blood pressure), people say that long waits are the second most common reason they switch physicians.

Patient Rx: Ask your doctor directly—not just the staff—what can be done to cut wait times. Try calling ahead to see if she's on schedule, or try morning visits, when the office may be less hectic. Finally, if long absences from work get you in trouble, ask the office to note on your chart, "Please see ASAP—must return to work." If these tactics fail, it may be time to switch physicians.

2. Be open to alternative medicine. More women than ever are turning to alternative remedies—and keeping it to themselves. (One study of women with breast cancer found that 46 percent kept mum about treatments.) Withholding any information can be dangerous because some herbs, for example, can hinder blood clotting. And St. John's wort affects the absorption of many drugs, says Susan Smolinske, PharmD, a toxicologist with the Children's Hospital of Michigan's Poison Control Center.

Patient Rx: If you are among the 62 percent of Americans who use alt med, tell your doctor. Say something as simple as "I've been going to an acupuncturist to help me, and I just wanted you to know," suggests Christine Brass-Jones, DO, an ob/gyn and director of the Center for True Harmony Wellness and Medicine in Mesa, Arizona. And ask a new doc if she prescribes alt meds—patients are most likely to confide in such physicians.

3. Ask me about my sex life. Even though sexual issues can signal larger health problems—including thyroid disorders, depression, STDs, and hormonal changes—doctors and patients balk at the topic. It's no wonder: A 2002 study from the University of North Carolina at Chapel Hill found that 35 percent of the nearly 1,000 women surveyed said that when they asked about libido, STDs, and other sexual heath concerns, even ob/gyns "seemed embarrassed by the subject," says Margaret Nusbaum, DO, MPH, a professor at UNC and lead author of the study.

Patient Rx: In a perfect world, your doctor would chat about sex at every visit, opening the door to potentially life-saving conversations. But if he doesn't respond to your concerns the first time, Dr. Nusbaum suggests placing your question in the context of a larger health issue. Say, "I am concerned about thyroid problems because my interest in sex has dwindled" or "Could my birth control pills be causing my vaginal dryness?" Still getting brushed off? Try this: "Whom would you refer me to in order to address this in greater detail?"

4. Understand I don't have insurance, but I'm too embarrassed to tell you. One in three Americans under 65 is without health insurance, including many in working families. Their ranks are swelling, drastically affecting preventive care.

Patient Rx: Level with your doctor because most want to help: In 2003, 65 percent of internists reduced fees or worked out payment plans for patients who lost their coverage, reports the New York Academy of Medicine. Ask if an adjustment can be made. Even if he says no, "doctors can steer you to many community programs that offer preventive services, such as mammograms, that most private-pay clients would never know about," says Charlie Shafer, MD, director of the Sioux River Valley Community Health Center in Sioux Falls, South Dakota.

5. Ask me about drug coverage, too, before you write a prescription. Not everyone who has health care coverage also has drug insurance, and drug coverage doesn't necessarily apply to all medications. "I had a patient whom I put on a cholesterol-lowering medication," says Dr. Shafer, "and I had her come back 3 months later for a retest. The results were bad, and she said, 'I never filled the prescription—I just couldn't afford it.'" In fact, only 35 percent of doctors are likely to ask patients about out-of-pocket costs, including medications, reports the Robert Wood Johnson Foundation.

Patient Rx: Ask if a generic is available: A month's worth of Lipitor can be $20 to $40—more expensive than the generic lovastatin. And don't worry that by asking for a generic you'll be missing out on some new, improved treatment; 78 percent of the drugs introduced between 1998 and 2003 are no better than those that were already on the market, according to Marcia Angell, MD, author of *The Truth About the Drug Companies.*

6. Use words I can understand, not medical jargon. The average medical school student learns between 5,000 and 10,000 new words in the first 2 years of medical school, says Dr. Lipkin. And jargon can put a patient at risk if, for example, a doctor discusses your "myocardial insufficiency" and you leave without even realizing he was referring to your weak heart. The Institute of Medicine reports that nearly half of all adults in the United States don't understand the health care information doctors give them, from prescriptions to follow-up schedules. Those people are more likely to be hospitalized and to require emergency services because they didn't follow directions.

Patient Rx: Besides the simple request to "say it in plain English, doc," it helps to have a second set of ears in the room. So if you know you're going to have an information-intensive visit (issues such as high blood pressure, asthma, or biopsy results all require more instruction than most mortals can absorb in one visit), bring along a friend or your spouse to help you remember what gets discussed, suggests Jacquelyn Ater, a Rochester, New York–based heath care coach who helps patients communicate with their doctors.

Better yet: Spend $40 on a small tape recorder so you can replay the discussion. Also ask your physician for Web site recommendations where you can find reliable research on your condition. Finally, ask if you can follow up by e-mail or phone or through a nurse if you have additional questions.

7. Say if you can't help me or tell me who can. Judy Soifer, 49, of Mill Valley, California, struggled with severe migraines most of her life. As they got worse, so did her physical dependence on painkilling narcotics—first, Demerol; later, Vicodin. "Over a 6-year period, I'd ask my neurologist if I could come off the Vicodin, and he'd say he didn't have any other drug that he thought could help me," she recounts. Finally, her doctor suggested that she travel to the Michigan Headache and Neurological Institute. Within weeks, Soifer was off narcotics and on newer medicine that helped control the headaches.

Patient Rx: If you have a chronic health problem, ask your doctor how long it will take to determine a new treatment's effectiveness and what comes next if it fails. If she suggests a different medication, ask how long it should take before you see results, and then follow up. Ask if you should schedule an appointment for that date or whether a phone consultation will work. If the answers aren't concrete or you simply have doubts about your treatment options, tell your doctor you want a second opinion—and don't worry that you're hurting her feelings, says Dr. Lipkin.

"Say, 'After I discussed this with my family, I feel it would be sensible to get a second opinion. Would you please arrange to provide Dr. _____ with copies of all my records?'" Second opinions for serious procedures are now the norm and are covered by insurance.

8. Give me a minute after you deliver a devastating diagnosis, then tell me what to do. Delivering bad news is a daily requirement for doctors, and some can be brutally matter-of-fact about it. "When a patient comes in with a symptom of frequent urination and the doctor diagnoses diabetes, to the doctor, that's routine. Sometimes we come across as uninterested," explains Dr. Lipkin. "But for the patient, it's a life-changing diagnosis." Doctors can convey that boredom, he says, by saying exactly the wrong thing ("This is common for your age") or multitasking (checking your chart when she should be giving you plenty of reassuring eye contact).

Patient Rx: Whether the bad news is huge (infertility or cancer) or small (no scuba diving this year), a recent Canadian study found that—after having empathy and privacy—people responded best to bad news when doctors quickly gave them the information they needed to take the next step. So when you've had a chance to compose yourself, ask your doctor for more information or to repeat himself if necessary. Load up on any free brochures, and ask him to jot down the titles of books he finds especially helpful (saving you an hour of paralysis at the bookstore), suggests Ater. Then find out if you need to see a medical specialist and how and when to follow up with him or a nurse in his practice.

9. Ask me if I'm feeling blue. The good news about depression is that doctors are trying to make sure this common problem is treated more effectively. In 2002, the US Preventive Services Task Force began asking all physicians to screen patients for depression with a simple two-question test. The bad news is that 50 percent of depression still goes undetected by primary care doctors, reports the Cleveland Clinic.

Patient Rx: It stinks that patients should have to be the ones to bring up depression, as Porras did, but that's the current reality. Call your doctor if you feel blue frequently; notice any change in sleep patterns, weight, or energy levels; or become irritable, weepy, or fatigued. Depression, twice as common in women as in men, causes misery, is associated with suicide, and has been linked to stroke, heart disease, and cancer. (For an online screening, go to www.depression-screening.org.)

10. At least glance at my chart before you give me advice. If you ever get the impression that your doctor is confusing you with another patient, you're not alone. "I'm a competitive triathlete, so when I had my hysterectomy, I had long conversations with my doctor about how the surgery would affect my training," says Star Walters, 52, of Salisbury Mills, New York. "At the second post-op visit, he told me I could start running again. Weeks later, when I went for the third visit, the doctor said, 'Okay, you can run now.'

"My husband panicked: 'But doc, she's already doing 9-milers!'" Walters was furious and wondered if her doctor had given her the green light to run by mistake. When such errors involve advice about diet or drug changes, the results can be life threatening.

Patient Rx: Patient overload is a growing problem for primary care doctors, who typically see or consult with 153 patients a week. Try starting each visit with "I don't mind if you take a few minutes to review my chart," suggests Abraham Verghese, MD, director of the

Center for Medical Humanities and Ethics at the University of Texas HSC at San Antonio. And if you do get the feeling that your doc's attention is elsewhere, speak up: "I notice you seem to remember less about me from visit to visit. Has there been a change in your caseload?" Dr. Verghese says this is a polite way to help him realize how inattentive he's being.

PATIENT, PLEASE . . .

1. Come with a list of questions, and warn me if you'll need extra time. Start with the biggest concerns first. Some patients ask for back-to-back appointments (and may be charged accordingly), though the last slot of the day may also give you more time with your doctor.

2. Understand if I'm grumpy. Some days, I don't like my job. Sure, you can dump a glum doctor, but talk to her first, suggests Barry Egener, MD, director of the Foundation for Medical Excellence in Portland, Oregon. "Say, 'I may be off base here, but I feel like something has changed in our interactions.' It might be the wake-up call she needs."

3. Don't be offended by sensitive questions. No, I don't think you look like a drug addict, a battered wife, or a sex machine. Doctors are supposed to ask patients about all kinds of embarrassing, high-risk behaviors because it does save lives (and remains confidential). So don't hold back.

4. Realize that we need to talk about your weight. Though two-thirds of all Americans weigh more than they should, it still is hard for doctors to say, "You're packing on the pounds." Rather than getting offended, get on the scale so you and your doctor can candidly discuss your risk for obesity-related illnesses such as cancer, heart disease, and diabetes.

5. Use the medicine exactly as prescribed—no freelance dosing. Half of all prescription drugs are taken incorrectly, according to a study by Cutting Edge Information, a pharmaceutical consult-

ing company. Have your doctor explain each prescription and why you need it. It's also a good idea to ask your pharmacist to go over the instructions so you can follow them to the letter.

6. Understand that figuring out what's covered is your job, not mine. Read your insurance plan guidelines and learn the usual coverage for the most commonly ordered tests: x-rays, ultrasounds, basic blood tests, and EKGs. And check in with your doctor's office manager, who may be more familiar with your plan.

7. Be patient. I don't like making you wait for specialty care either. If you need to see a specialist, ask your primary care physician for several referrals, not just one. That way you can find a specialist who fits with your needs and time frame.

MEDICAL BREAKTHROUGHS

Here's the latest and greatest diabetes research to help you take control.

BE A FORTUNE-TELLER

Figure out your health future for free: Log on to www.diabetes.org/phd for Diabetes PHD (Personal Health Decisions), a new risk assessment tool. Plug in information such as weight, blood pressure, and cholesterol, and the program will crunch your odds for diabetes, heart attack, and more, based on clinical research.

DIG INTO YOUR PAST

There's more hanging on the family tree than your good looks: Researchers have discovered a variant gene that may cause diabetes, according to a study in the journal *Nature Genetics*. Scientists analyzed the genetic records of 3,774 people and found that 38 percent of them carried a copy of TCFL2, a gene that may disrupt insulin function. Another 7 percent had two copies—meaning they'd inherited it from both parents. One copy of the gene increased diabetes risk by 45 percent; two copies increased risk by 140 percent, says study author Kari Stefansson, MD. A test for the gene should be available in about 3 years.

In another study, scientists at Saint Louis University zeroed in on a gene variant responsible for raising a person's risk of type 2 diabetes. According to the study, people with Ala54Thr absorb and burn fat more quickly after a meal, which may slow the removal of sugar from their blood. The finding could lead to new gene-based diabetes drugs.

SNOOZE AWAY DIABETES RISK

Shortchanging yourself on shut-eye has serious consequences. A Boston University study revealed that too little sleep may raise your diabetes risk.

Researchers asked 1,486 people about their sleep habits, then took blood samples to measure glucose tolerance. Folks who logged fewer than 5 hours of sack time were $2^1/_2$ times more likely to have diabetes than people who slept for 7 or 8 hours. Lack of sleep triggers the release of fatty acids, forcing insulin to work overtime to clear them away, says study author Daniel Gottlieb, MD.

NURSE FOR BETTER GLUCOSE LEVELS

Breastfeeding can reduce a woman's risk of developing type 2 diabetes, according to a study in the *Journal of the American Medical Association*. Researchers studied 157,003 women and found that breastfeeding for at least a year reduced a woman's risk of developing the disease by as much as 15 percent.

"Nursing moms have lower glucose and insulin levels," explains study author Alison Mann Stuebe, MD. "These hormonal changes over a long period of nursing may translate into a lower diabetes risk."

The findings were cumulative: If you have two kids, breastfeed each for 6 months to get the same benefit; breastfeed each for a year and you'll double your protection.

CHECK THE STATE OF YOUR PATE

Young men with thinning hair are at greater risk of diabetes, according to a new study. Researchers at the Institute of Endocrinology in Prague analyzed the blood of two dozen men and found that those who began balding before age 30 were more likely to be insulin resistant—raising their risk of diabetes—than men with hair to spare. Tests also revealed that as the baldies' levels of follicle-stimulating hormone decreased, their insulin resistance increased, meaning a hormone deficiency may have been at work.

Men who see scalp in their twenties should get a fasting blood glucose test:

Levels over 100 milligrams per deciliter signal trouble.

STAY OUT OF THE HOME

If bingo, shuffleboard, and pureed prunes don't tickle your fancy, listen up: How you live now can influence where you live later, say Rutgers University researchers. For 20 years, they tracked 3,526 adults ages 45 to 64. After checking for smoking, activity, weight gain, blood pressure, and diabetes incidence, they found that an early diagnosis of type 2 diabetes more than tripled a person's chance of ending up in a nursing home.

Smoking increased the likelihood by 56 percent, inactivity by 40 percent, and high blood pressure by 35 percent. Even more debilitating: The combination of diabetes plus any of the other risk factors increased the odds of admission fourfold.

To keep a rest-home stay out of your future, study coauthor Louise Russell, PhD, recommends quitting smoking, exercising regularly, and maintaining a healthy weight—starting today. "The risk of being sent to a nursing home—and the opportunity to avoid it—begins in early middle age," she says.

TUNE IN YOUR RADAR

Women have more diabetes warning signs, say University of Buffalo researchers. They studied healthy adults and found that markers of inflammation, as well as poor blood clotting, ID'd women—but not men—who would become prediabetic.

MIND YOUR MOOD

The next time you order the pancake platter, pay close attention: Feeling cranky or forgetful after a high-carb breakfast is an indicator of prediabetes.

In a study, UK researchers had people eat a carb-loaded meal—the equivalent of two diner flapjacks or a large bagel—first thing in the morning. Then they monitored the participants' memory and mood for nearly 2 hours afterward. The finding: Those who exhibited the poorest recall and attitude also had the greatest fluctuations in blood sugar, an early warning sign of diabetes.

If these symptoms sound familiar or you find yourself feeling sluggish after eating carbohydrates, ask your doctor for a glucose tolerance test. It's one of the earliest ways of catching diabetes before it takes hold.

TAKE THIS TEST

Doctors will soon be able to tell if you're on the road to diabetes simply by shining a light on your forearm—a painless test that takes only 1 minute. Scout, a device manufactured by VeraLight, emits a beam that measures collagen changes and the amount of blood sugar by-products hiding out in your skin. A high reading means your body likely isn't processing glucose efficiently—a hallmark of the disease, explains John Maynard, VeraLight vice president of product development.

The test could have big benefits. Right now, diabetes screenings involve an overnight fast and having blood drawn the next day. But Scout could be used on the spot during a regular checkup, even if you downed a plate of waffles for breakfast. It ups the chance of catching the disease earlier, when it is more easily treated, which may help you avoid complications such as kidney problems.

The device won't be available until 2008, but you can take action now: Assess your risk of developing the dis-ease by logging on to www.diabetes.org/risk-test. And continue getting screened the usual way by your doctor, too.

EASIER DIABETES CONTROL

Two-thirds of the nation's diabetics don't have their blood sugar under control. A new tool makes it much easier to keep tabs: The Guardian REAL-Time Continuous Glucose Monitoring System gives regular readings—no finger pricks needed.

Here's how it works: A tiny sensor is inserted beneath the skin at the waist. It records sugar levels, sending readings every 5 minutes to a monitor clipped to your pants. If glucose levels get too high or low, the monitor will vibrate (or beep). Ask your doctor about it, or visit www.minimed.com for more info.

GUM UP SOME DIABETES PROTECTION

Brush, floss, and call the dentist if you have type 2 diabetes. Surprising research suggests that TLC for your gums could cut blood sugar—and your risk of diabetic complications such as heart disease, stroke, blindness, and kidney failure.

In the study, 20 women and men ages 35 to 70 with periodontal disease—gum infection and inflammation that can be triggered by poor dental hygiene—received a common treatment called scaling and root planing. The 10 volunteers with diabetes got a bonus: When tested 6 months after treatment had ended, their average blood sugar levels had dropped by as much as 20 percent, report researchers from Madrid's Complutense University.

The link? Infected gums can flood the bloodstream with immune system compounds, including a substance called tumor necrosis factor (TNF), which interferes with the ability of cells to absorb blood sugar. If you have diabetes, good dental hygiene and regular checkups are a must.

CONSIDER THIS SUPPLEMENT

Could an herb called fenugreek be the answer to high blood sugar?

People with type 2 diabetes who took 1 gram of fenugreek seed extract for 2 months reduced their blood sugar lev-

els by about 20 percent—the same amount as those who followed a standard nutrition and exercise program, a small study in India found.

If you take it, continue managing your condition with medication, activity, and a healthy diet. "It's safe for most people," says Ryan Bradley, ND, head of the Diabetes and Cardiovascular Wellness Program at the Bastyr Center for Natural Health. (Follow label instructions; do not take fenugreek if you're on blood thinners.)

Fenugreek may be a helpful addition to your diabetes treatment plan, but talk with your doc before you begin taking it on your own.

BOOST DIABETES CONTROL AT WORK

Getting your blood sugar under control may be easier when the boss is involved. In the first study of its kind, Brigham Young University scientists asked 35 employees—31 were prediabetic, 4 diabetic—of a local company to stick with a yearlong wellness program held at the office. Before, during, and after work they attended classes on nutrition and exercise, and they had free access to an on-site nurse. They were also encouraged to do a 30-minute workout daily.

After 6 months, participants showed remarkable improvement: Their blood glucose levels dropped by 25 percent; their weight fell by 6 pounds, on average; and they trimmed more than an inch from their waistlines. Red flags such as high cholesterol, triglycerides, and blood pressure decreased as well. After 12 months, 18 of the prediabetics had reached normal, healthy status, and 3 of the 4 people with diabetes were free of the disease.

The workplace is good for reinforcing lifestyle changes, says lead researcher Steven Aldana, PhD, partly because it makes it easy for employees to attend helpful classes: "It's a great support system."

ASK THESE QUESTIONS

Your doc may be holding back critical info when she hands you that prescription. When University of California researchers eavesdropped on 44 physicians who doled out prescriptions to 185 patients, they exposed a glaring communication gap: Doctors neglected to mention potential side effects 65 percent of the time. In 66 percent of cases, they didn't tell patients how long to take a new drug, and details on how often to take meds were left out in 42 percent of conversations.

"Lack of information could cause a patient to miss signs that a drug is causing more harm than good—or even overdose," notes lead study author Derjung M. Tarn, MD, PhD, an assistant professor of family medicine at the David Geffen School of Medicine at UCLA. When you get an Rx, be sure to ask your doctor or your pharmacist these crucial questions.

1. When and for how long should I take this drug?
2. Are there any side effects, and what should I do if I experience them?
3. Are there any foods, beverages, medications, or herbal supplements I should avoid while taking this?
4. What should I do if I miss a dose?

Success Story

She Won't Let Diabetes Slow Her Down

Jean Jennings is a globe-trotting, fast-driving automotive journalist who has friends, family, and a career that she loves. She doesn't have time to deal with diabetes, she says.

Jean quit smoking cold turkey one October day 10 years ago, after a particularly aggressive intervention by friends. She didn't want to gain the 10 pounds that always pile on when you quit, so she decided to give up deep-fried onion rings (her favorite vegetable) and beer (her favorite grain).

It worked. Jean stopped smoking, and she didn't gain the 10 pounds. In fact, after a month without beer and grease, she actually lost a few pounds. Soon she was 20 pounds down and then 30. Jean gradually began sampling the forbidden fries and a brew or two. But the weight continued to fall. Soon, she was back to her usual happy oblivion of fast food and tall beers. By that spring, after a lifetime of being heftier than your average girly girl, she had dropped an inexplicable 70 pounds from her nearly 6-foot frame.

And then the inexplicable was explained.

Jean needed a physical to renew her car-racing license, and she went to a doctor who would sign off without scrutinizing her too closely. Sure enough, he just made her look at the eye chart, pee in a cup, and give him advice on how to improve the performance of his Porsche. She left with the paperwork signed. But the doctor called that afternoon with startling news. "Sugar," he said to Jean, "you've got sugar."

"Diabetes? There must be some mistake" thought Jean. Sure, her dad had developed diabetes in childhood. But she was 43 years old. This was not her father's kind of diabetes, however; it was the type that has to do with obesity, a bad diet, and inactivity. "Oh, wait. That all applies to me," Jean thought.

(continued)

Success Story (cont.)

And so began what remains today, 10 years on, the most frightening, aggravating, inscrutable, and never-ending battle of Jean's life. She learned she had diabetes and, no, there was no mistake. "Your sugar registered so high in the urine specimen that we don't need to do a fasting test," she was told. "Have you been getting up in the night to pee?"

"I suppose I have," Jean said.

"Have you been exhausted?"

"Yes, but I write for a car magazine and fly more than 100,000 miles a year. I never sit down," Jean replied.

"Didn't you think it was weird that you lost 70 pounds on the cheeseburger, onion rings, and beer diet?"

"I thought it was a late-in-life gift from God."

It was Jean's typical smart-aleck remark. She loved her full-tilt, boogying life; healthy food and exercise were never high on her list of priorities. She knew there would be consequences at some point, but she never expected to develop diabetes. Some gift. Now she had to take care of herself. "Oh well," she decided. "Let's have at it."

Jean became instantly and insanely compliant, with a level of obsessiveness that a Marine would have had a tough time maintaining. She couldn't, either. The change was just too severe, and she missed living the good life. There is apparently a predictable progression for people with chronic illness that goes something like: I Can Beat This, I Hate This (and All of You), Maybe I Don't Really Have This, and so on, until they either pull themselves together or they die. Jean marched right through to stage three and then ran out of steam. A mere 6 months after her diagnosis, she gave up on the healthy diet, drifted away from the gym, and started to regain the weight. Soon she'd put back on all 70 pounds.

Jean was doing okay on her blood tests, though, because she was taking a drug medication called Rezulin (troglitazone). Unfortunately, her miracle drug was suddenly pulled off the market because of a pesky little side effect: It could destroy the liver.

Now Jean was in trouble. Fatter than she had ever been (the clinical term is "obese") and lacking any eating or exercise discipline, she could no longer keep her blood sugar in check. Jean didn't want to inject insulin—using a needle would mean that she really, truly did have diabetes and that she'd failed to control it on her own. But as her doctor tried to find a blood sugar–lowering pill as effective as Rezulin, her blood sugar shot sky-high. Jean went nearly blind for a couple of weeks as the sugar in her system literally changed the prismatic effect in her eyes. Jean's husband drove her to and from the office. One day, she had to deliver a speech to a roomful of people she couldn't see. She was absolutely terrified. Luckily, it was a temporary vision loss that cleared up once the new drugs got the excess sugar out of her bloodstream.

By the time Jean had been struggling with diabetes for 4 long years, the idea that the disease presented her with the opportunity to get healthy had faded to a distant memory. Jean knew she could produce a dramatic drop in glucose readings by eating sensibly and walking 30 minutes a day. Only she just couldn't do it.

Truth be told, Jean still had no real idea of the damage diabetes was doing inside of her. Then her beloved Aunt Red went into a diabetic coma. The doctor in intensive care said her leg was infected and she needed to have it amputated. When Jean asked why he didn't put a stent or something in her leg to help her circulation, he just looked at her. "You don't get it, do you?" he asked. "I can't put a stent in. The high sugar has exploded her capillaries. Those vessels are mush." Jean knew she would take that image with her forever—of what diabetes had done to her aunt, and what it was doing to herself.

Jean finally got herself a new endocrinologist, who checked her 3-month average blood sugar and immediately informed her that her oral drugs weren't doing the job; Jean had to go on insulin.

(continued)

Success Story (cont.)

"Why are you crying?" the doctor asked Jean the first time she pressed a syringe to her stomach and injected.

"I am a failure," Jean said, sobbing.

The doctor looked a little puzzled. "You're not a bad person," she told Jean. "You just have a bad pancreas."

Jean has a different image of diabetes now. It's not a gift, and it's not a punishment. "It's like rust in the engine of one of the cars I drive, and unless I watch out, it will corrode the pipes and blow the gaskets," Jean says.

So here's the perfect ending to the story: Jean is joining Weight Watchers, and she's started swimming at the YMCA. She's taken on the dog-walking duty for the household, and it's turned into one of the most delightful parts of her hectic day.

Now here's the real ending: Every day, Jean gets up and hopes to God that she does just one of those things. And every 3 months, she sees her chief mechanic: her endocrinologist, who adjusts her meds, gives her encouragement, and sends her back on the road.

"This is the best I can do at living right so my disease doesn't kill me—while living well so my disease doesn't steal everything I love about my life," Jean says. "I like to drive cars fast. I'll slow down on the curves if I have to, but nobody's going to take away my keys."

Part II

EAT RIGHT

CHAPTER 6

THE DIABETES DIET

The new approach to eating well

It may sound strange, but there's never been a better time to have diabetes. Gone are the days when a doctor handed you a list of what you could and couldn't eat—the same list he gave to everyone else who came in the door. New evidence has significantly altered the one-size-fits-all dietary approach to this condition.

For example, even though it's best to eat sugar in moderation (and not just if you have diabetes), for most people with diabetes, it's no longer forbidden. Some may be advised to cut back on fat and eat more carbohydrates; others will be told just the opposite. In fact, it's not unusual these days for two people with diabetes, even if they are the same age, same weight, and in the same overall condition, to have totally different diets for controlling it.

Yet one aspect of diabetes has stayed the same. Diet—what you eat and, in some cases, what you don't—is at the heart of any treatment plan. Along with maintaining a healthy weight and getting regular exercise, eating right helps keep blood sugar and fats at steady levels, which is the key to keeping problems under control.

HUNGER AMID PLENTY

Before seeing how you can use food to treat or prevent diabetes, here's a quick refresher on what this condition is. The fuel that keeps our bodies running is sugar. Doctors call it glucose. Soon after we eat, glucose pours into the bloodstream and is carried to individual cells throughout the body. Before it can enter these cells, however, it requires the presence of a hormone called insulin. And therein lies the problem.

People with diabetes either don't produce enough insulin or the insulin they do produce doesn't work efficiently. In either case, all that glucose in the bloodstream isn't able to get inside the cells. Rather, it hovers in the bloodstream, getting more and more concentrated as time goes by. Not only do individual cells go hungry, which can cause fatigue, dizziness, and many other symptoms, but all that concentrated sugar becomes toxic, eventually damaging the eyes, kidneys, nerves, immune system, heart, and blood vessels.

The more serious form of diabetes—and, fortunately, the less common—is type 1, or insulin-dependent, diabetes. It occurs when the body makes little or no insulin of its own. People with type 1 diabetes must take insulin in order to replace their own missing supplies.

Far more common is type 2, or non-insulin-dependent, diabetes. People with this condition—which occurs mainly in those over age 40 but is becoming more and more common in younger people, even kids—produce some insulin but generally not enough. They may take oral medications but generally don't require insulin injections, at least not in the early stages of the disease.

THE HEALING POWER OF FOOD

Experts have long recognized that what you eat can play a critical role both in preventing and controlling type 2 diabetes. Perhaps the best way to understand the effects of diet on diabetes is to look at two similar groups of people who differ primarily in what they eat.

Consider the Pima Indians. Researchers discovered that Pimas who live in Mexico and eat a lot of corn, beans, and fruits are seldom overweight and rarely develop diabetes. By contrast, the Pima

Indians in Arizona eat an American-ized diet that is high in sugar and fat. They commonly develop diabetes by age 50.

HEALING FIBER

A high-fiber diet has been shown to relieve everything from constipation to heart disease. Research suggests that it can also play a powerful role in control-ling blood sugar, says James W. Ander-son, MD, professor of internal medicine in the department of endocrinology and molecular medicine at the University of Kentucky in Lexington.

There are two types of fiber: soluble and insoluble. Both play a role in stabi-lizing blood sugar.

Here's how soluble fiber helps: Because it forms a gummy gel in the intestine, soluble fiber helps prevent glucose from being absorbed into the blood too quickly. This in turn helps keep blood sugar levels from rising or dipping too drastically.

In addition, soluble fiber seems to increase cells' sensitivity to insulin, so

Toss One Back

Beer is probably the last thing you'd expect to be on a diabetes-friendly diet. But researchers at Boston Medical Center found that mild to moderate alcohol con-sumption—of beer and wine, specifically—was associated with a lower risk of hyperinsulinemia (having too much insulin in the blood, which is often associ-ated with diabetes). The people in the study who drank 20 drinks per month were 66 percent less likely to be diagnosed with an obesity-related condition, such as diabetes, than those who abstained.

Don't look at this as a license to binge, however, and talk with your doctor before adding alcohol to your diabetes diet. Safe upper limits are one drink per day for women and two for men. A drink is defined as 12 ounces of beer, 5 ounces of wine, or $1^1/_2$ ounces of liquor.

more sugar can move from the blood into the cells.

In studies conducted by Dr. Anderson, people with type 2 diabetes who ate a high-fiber (and high-carbohydrate) diet were able to improve their blood sugar control by an average of 95 percent. People with type 1 diabetes on the same diet showed a 30 percent improvement.

Research now shows that insoluble fiber may play a role in diabetes prevention as well. Insoluble fiber is found in whole grain products, vegetables such as green beans and dark green leafy vegetables, fruit skins and root vegetable skins, seeds, and nuts. In a study conducted at Harvard University, averaging 10 grams of cereal fiber each day (from foods such as whole grain breads, rice, and pasta) lowered the risk of type 2 diabetes by 36 percent.

It's really very easy to increase your fiber intake. Try eating at least five servings of fruits and vegetables each day. Eat more whole grain bread. (The first ingredient should be 100 percent whole wheat flour or stone-ground whole wheat flour. Another clue is that the bread should provide $1\,^1/_2$ to 2 grams of fiber per slice. Don't be fooled by just a brown color, which can simply be molasses!)

Use whole grain cereals and whole wheat pasta instead of white pasta. And swap out beans for meat in some meals.

You don't have to be fanatical about counting fiber grams. You can easily get enough by eating 3 to 5 servings of vegetables, 2 to 4 servings of fruits, and 6 to 11 servings of breads, cereals, pasta, and rice a day.

Two great sources of fiber are Brussels sprouts and beans. A half-cup serving of Brussels sprouts contains 4 grams of fiber, with 2 grams of soluble fiber. (That's more fiber than you'll get in a cup of pasta.) A half-cup of kidney beans contains nearly 7 grams of fiber, almost 3 grams of it soluble.

Increase your fiber intake slowly to avoid some uncomfortable digestive issues, and drink more water to help keep the fiber moving through your system.

HELP FROM VITAMINS

Perhaps it's appropriate that vitamin D is helpful for diabetes. Researchers at Tufts University in Boston discovered that getting enough of the sunshine vitamin (so-called because your body makes vitamin D from time spent in the sun) may help reduce the risk of type 2 diabetes. The scientists studied 81,700 women for 20 years and found that the women who had the highest intake of vitamin D (which you can get not only from being out in the sun but also from foods) had a 28 percent lower risk of type 2 diabetes than the women who had the lowest intake of vitamin D.

Possibly the easiest way to get vitamin D in your diet is by drinking fortified milk. Having one glass of fortified milk will provide about 100 IU, or 25 percent of the Daily Value (DV) for this vitamin. Another great reason to do that is because you'll also get milk's calcium. One cup of fat-free milk contains more than 300 milligrams of calcium, which is almost a third of the DV for this mineral.

Why is calcium important for people with type 2 diabetes? It's also key in the fight against this disease. When Harvard scientists studied the diets of more than 41,000 men for 12 years, they found that for every daily serving of low-fat dairy foods the men ate each day, their risk of developing type 2 diabetes dropped by 9 percent. The researchers think that the calcium in low-fat dairy plays a role.

But probably the best strategy is to get both vitamin D and calcium together,

and, of course, you can get that combo in one convenient package: a carton of milk. Researchers at Tufts–New England Medical Center in Boston found that among the 83,779 women studied, those who got the highest levels of both vitamin D and calcium had a 33 percent lower risk of type 2 diabetes than the women who got the least. How high was that highest level? More than 1,200 milligrams of calcium each day and more than 800 IU of vitamin D.

Two other important vitamins for diabetes care are C and E. In fact, if you have diabetes, fruits and vegetables rich in vitamins C and E may be your ticket to healthier eyes, nerves, and blood vessels. These vitamins are known as antioxidants. They help protect your body's cells from free radicals, naturally occurring, cell-damaging molecules that may pose particular risks to people with diabetes.

What's more, vitamin C may provide even more direct benefits. In one study, Italian researchers gave 40 people with diabetes 1 gram of vitamin C every day. After 4 months, the patients' abilities to use insulin had significantly improved, perhaps because vitamin C helps insulin penetrate cells.

The DV for vitamin C is 60 milligrams.

Oranges and grapefruit are excellent sources of vitamin C, but they're not the only ones. One cup of chopped, steamed broccoli, for example, contains more than 116 milligrams, or almost twice the DV for vitamin C. Half a cantaloupe has about 113 milligrams of vitamin C, and one red bell pepper has 140 milligrams.

Even though vitamin C is essential for people with diabetes, this nutrient is readily destroyed during cooking. For example, boiled broccoli may retain only 45 percent of its vitamin C. Steaming, which can preserve 70 percent of the C, is better. Best of all is microwaving, which preserves as much as 85 percent.

Another way to increase your intake of vitamin C is to pick the ripest fruits. Scarlet tomatoes, garnet strawberries, and deep chartreuse kiwifruit are much more nutrient-dense than fruits that haven't yet hit their prime.

Vitamin E, which is good for the heart, may be particularly important for people with diabetes, who are two to three times more likely to develop heart disease than people who do not have the disease. And research suggests that, like vitamin C, vitamin E may help insulin work better.

Finnish scientists studied 944 men and found that those with the lowest levels of vitamin E in their blood were four times more likely to have diabetes than those with the highest levels. Vitamin E may somehow help insulin carry sugar from the blood into cells in muscles and tissues, the researchers speculate.

Vitamin E also helps keep blood platelets, which are elements in blood that help it clot, from becoming too sticky. This is particularly important in people with diabetes, whose platelets tend to clump more readily and lead to heart disease.

To get an adequate amount of vitamin E, you need to occasionally use oils rich in polyunsaturated fats, like soybean oil, corn oil, and sunflower oil. Of course, these oils don't provide the benefits of the monounsaturated fats found in olive oil and canola oil. Used in moderation, however, they will help boost your vitamin E to healthy levels.

Wheat germ is another excellent source of vitamin E, with a quarter cup containing 6 IU, or 20 percent of the DV. Other good sources of this vitamin include kale, sweet potatoes, almonds, avocados, and blueberries.

CHROME-PLATED PROTECTION

It's not just vitamins that can help control diabetes. The trace mineral chromium, found in broccoli, grapefruit, and fortified breakfast cereals, has been shown to improve the body's ability to regulate blood sugar, says Richard A. Anderson, PhD, a research chemist with the USDA Human Nutrition Research Center in Beltsville, Maryland.

Tests show that people with diabetes have lower levels of chromium circulating in their blood than people without the disease. In one study, eight people who had difficulty regulating blood sugar were given 20 micrograms of chromium a day. After 5 weeks, their blood sugar levels fell by as much as 50 percent. People without blood sugar problems who were given chromium showed no such change.

In two studies, scientists found that chromium may help control the health risks of diabetes. In one study, researchers studied 27 people with diabetes for 10 months and found that insulin sensitivity was twice as good in the people who took chromium as in people who took a fake supplement. Another study, this one in Slovenia, found that in people with diabetes, taking chromium supplements for 3 months shortened QTc intervals, which is a heart rhythm that may become fatal if the interval lengthens.

It's true that the people in these studies took chromium supplements. But because experts aren't sure that taking chromium supplements is safe, it's best to boost your supplies of this trace mineral by eating foods that provide it. One cup of broccoli, for example, contains 22 micrograms, or 18 percent of the DV. A 2 1/2-ounce waffle has almost 7 micrograms, 6 percent of the DV. And 1 cup of grape juice contains 8 micrograms, or 6 percent of the DV.

When you're trying to get more chromium, barley is a good choice. One animal study done in England found that barley can help keep blood sugar levels under control. This grain makes great soups and breads and is a nice addition to casseroles.

To help your body retain the most chromium, it's helpful to eat plenty of complex carbohydrates, such as pasta and bagels, says Dr. Anderson. Eating lots of sugary foods, on the other hand, will cause your body to excrete chromium. So even though it's fine to enjoy an occasional sweet snack, the emphasis should really be on the healthier whole foods, he says.

The USDA recommends eating whole grains (such as whole wheat flour, whole wheat bread, and brown rice) instead of refined grains (such as white flour, white bread, and white rice) whenever possible. Whole grains provide many health benefits, in addition to helping your body retain chromium.

MAGNESIUM FOR GLUCOSE CONTROL

Experts estimate that 25 percent of people with diabetes are low in the mineral magnesium. The problem is even worse in those who have diabetes-related heart disease or a type of eye damage known as retinopathy. Since low levels of magnesium have been linked to damage to the retinas, it's likely that upping your intake of this mineral may help protect your eyes.

Good sources of magnesium include baked halibut, which contains 91 milligrams of magnesium per 3-ounce serving, or 23 percent of the DV. Cooked spinach is also good: One cup contains 157 milligrams, or almost 40 percent of the DV. And a half-cup serving of long-grain brown rice has 42 milligrams, 11 percent of the DV.

PUTTING IT ALL TOGETHER

Treating and preventing diabetes with foods involves more than just eating a few good foods. It's really a whole diet in which all the separate elements—fiber, vitamins, minerals, and so forth—are brought together in one good plan. You might consider working with a dietitian to develop a meal plan that promotes blood sugar control, coordinates with your medications, and is tailored to your individual preferences and lifestyle.

CHAPTER 7

EAT-RIGHT RULES THAT WORK

Eat, drink, and be healthy

Ever wonder what nutritionists eat? Get a glimpse inside the pantries of four top nutritionists as they share their real-world, study-backed tips.

LET YOUR CULTURE INSPIRE YOUR EATING HABITS

Kibbe Conti was working on South Dakota's Pine Ridge Indian Reservation when her nutrition education collided with her culture.

As a certified diabetes educator, she knew that rates of type 2 diabetes among Native Americans are more than two times the national average. As a Lakota Sioux well versed in her history, she also knew that their diets were once healthy—made up of gathered plants, quality meats, and fish. But when Indian land shrank to reservation size, highly processed meat products and soda replaced extralean buffalo meat and fresh water—not the best choices for people prone to obesity and diabetes, she says. Conti hopes to help by reintroducing more traditional foods into a diet plan that reflects how her ancestors ate: large game animals, fruits, and starchy vegetables.

In her own home, "I practice what I preach," says the 39-year-old mother of two. Instead of sweetened drinks, she sips water, milk, or seltzer, and her family eats lean meat—most of the time. "My husband is Italian, and he's from New York," she says. "He really likes sausage, so sometimes he has to have it."

My Diet Rules

Buy locally. "Our ancestors ate off the land they lived on, so we try our best to do the same. I pick up fresh fruits and vegetables at the market whenever they are available, and I keep organic milk and eggs on hand."

Make veggies your starch. "Native people used to eat beans, corn, and squash, which contain complex carbohydrates that gradually release glucose into your blood instead of spiking your blood sugar."

Shop slowly. "Our ancestors painstakingly hunted, gathered, and prepared food. These days, most of us spend almost no time. Slow down at the store, read the nutrition labels, peruse the fresh meat—healthy eating starts with healthy shopping."

HAVE DESSERT FIRST

Judith S. Stern, ScD, RD, teaches at the University of California, Davis. She also leads an international team of experts charged with establishing criteria by which the latest obesity research papers are evaluated.

"Chocolate should be an honorary vitamin," says Dr. Stern. Not the first thing you'd expect to hear from an obesity researcher, but in "real life," this 64-year-old is a pie-baking, freewheeling gourmet. She'll spread a little butter—guilt free—on her whole grain bread and often shares her daily oatmeal-and-raisin breakfast with her macaw, Papaya. And she doesn't apologize for the extra 20 pounds she carries on her petite frame. "I am happy with myself as I am," says Dr. Stern, whose blood pressure and cholesterol levels are well within the healthy range. "I just love food." (She has been known to snap a picture of a particularly good restaurant meal.) And sometimes she even eats dessert first. "Just thinking of chocolate makes me hum," she says, laughing. But so do fresh fruits and vegetables. Dr. Stern is just as rhapsodical when she talks about Italian plums, so much so that she makes them sound as tempting as tiramisu. "There's only one 'fruit' I don't like," she quips. "It's against my religion to eat rhubarb."

My Diet Rules

Think small but spectacular. "I'm very particular. I won't eat bad-tasting food just because it's there. I'd rather have smaller portions of something that tastes great."

Go au naturel. "I never put sugar on fruit—not because sugar is evil but because fruit is already so sweet. And I don't use salt. I appreciate the real taste of food, and adding anything else is just gilding the lily."

Make extra bites impossible. "None of us really have the visual judgment to estimate half a meal, so when I'm at a restaurant, I order an appetizer as my entrée, or I'll ask the server to bring me just half. My favorite restaurant is a Spanish tapas place that serves nothing but appetizers."

PASS UP THE WHITE STUFF

Cheryl Forberg, RD, author of *Stop the Clock! Cooking*, is the behind-the-scenes dietitian for NBC's *The Biggest Loser* reality TV show, and she helped contestants lose a combined total of more than 800 pounds.

To earn a spot in Forberg's pantry, a food has to be an edible version of an overachiever: rich in nutrients and tops in antioxidants. What you won't see anywhere in her Napa, California, kitchen is refined flour or sugar. "I don't cook with or eat either of them," says the 51-year-old chef. "They're nothing more than calories, so I don't make them part of my diet."

Peek in her fridge and you'll find vibrantly colored fruits and vegetables, such as pink grapefruit or spinach, and good protein sources such as fish, lean meat, and low-fat dairy. Comb the cabinets, and you'll see whole grains, nuts, seeds, and legumes. Through her research, she found that incorporating these types of foods into the diet not only helps fight disease but also helps prevent the effects of aging.

"The more I learned, the more I wondered why I would eat anything else," she says. "I felt better, and my skin looks better, too." In fact, Forberg is so committed to her food style that even her Boston terrier, Ben, eats the same healthy diet. "He loves salmon and spinach," she says.

My Diet Rules

Use "healthier" sugar. "I [always] cook with neutral-tasting agave nectar or sorghum syrup, which is high in antioxidants."

Bag a nutritious snack. "I pack a few handfuls of homemade granola in my pocketbook when I travel. It helps me avoid the easy airport or minibar temptations and provides an instant energy boost."

Forget fancy. "I'm as busy as anyone else, so I don't have time to make elaborate meals three times a day. Oatmeal speckled with fruit and nuts for breakfast, grilled chicken or fish over salad for dinner—those are my favorite and healthy 'fast foods.'"

SAVE ROOM FOR FUN

Claudia Gonzalez, RD, moved from Peru to Miami at age 19 and turned her interest in nutrition into a career devoted to fighting the rising obesity rate in the Latino community.

"If you don't eat right, neither will your children," she says. That's the first thing this pediatric dietitian tells the Latino families she counsels, and it's a belief that she follows at home with her own three kids.

Latino children have among the highest obesity rates in the United States, and Gonzalez works to help families take the first step toward change. "Some of my clients tell me they don't like vegetables, but if they don't eat them, it'll be difficult to convince their kids to," says Gonzalez, 41. You don't have to give up family favorites; the key is learning to blend traditional flavors into healthier meals. "You can have that fried chicken, for example, as long as half the plate is filled with something green," says Gonzalez, coauthor of *Gordito Doesn't Mean Healthy*, a Latino eating guide.

Another tip for Latina moms: Adopt your culture's definition of comfort. "Latin Americans associate the word *comfort* with friends, not food," says Gonzalez, who'd never heard the term "comfort food" until coming to the United States. "If you're feeling stressed, call a good girlfriend to walk or go shopping. That way you're moving, not eating."

My Diet Rules

Think in food groups. "At every meal, get two or three food groups—choose between whole grains, dairy, fruits and vegetables, and meat and fish. My son, for example, loves cereal, so he has it with milk and a banana, and my daughter might have her yogurt with a little fruit or a slice of whole wheat bread."

Always split dessert. "In our house, no one gets any kind of junk food or sweet to themselves. When a package is opened, it's shared."

Alternate heavy and light meals. "Sometimes if I don't have a really healthy lunch, I make up for it by making sure my dinner is better. As long as two out of three of my meals are packed with nutrients, I know I'm doing okay."

CHAPTER 8

THE DIABETES PROMOTER IN YOUR FRIDGE

It raises diabetes risk and robs bone. It's wrecking our teeth. And it's making us fat. The culprit? Soda

For most of her life, Abbey Arndt, 33, has been a soda addict.

In the middle of the morning, she'd indulge her first craving of the day with a trip to the office refrigerator to grab one of the free sodas her company supplied. Coca-Cola, Pepsi, Mountain Dew, cherry soda—it didn't matter; she was an equal-opportunity drinker. In the afternoon, she'd snatch another can, and dinner often meant a third. "If I wasn't drinking soda, I was thinking about it," says Arndt, a corporate consultant who lives in Grafton, Wisconsin.

Her weight problems began at age 10, soon after she began drinking large amounts of pop, and continued into her twenties and thirties. At her peak, she weighed 314 pounds. Besides feeling heavy and out of shape, she dealt with rampant cavities, frequent mood swings, and erratic energy levels: "I'd get lethargic midmorning, so I'd grab a soda, thinking it would give me a pick-me-up. I'd be a little hyper, but then half an hour later, I would practically be asleep at my keyboard."

Arndt's passion for pop is all too familiar to the average American, who drinks 18 ounces, or more than two full glasses, of soft drinks a day. In fact, according to a study in 2005, soda and other sugar-sweetened drinks have become the largest source of calories in the American diet, replacing white bread. The proliferation of soda tells the story. There are 450 different varieties sold in the United States. While soft drinks are still king, with sales reaching $68.1 billion in 2005, sports-drink sales have increased 19.3 percent over the past year, to $1.5 billion.

People may think they're doing something healthy "by grabbing a bottle of Powerade instead of a can of Coke," says Kara Gallagher, PhD, an assistant professor of exercise physiology at the University of Louisville and a *Prevention* advisor. But at 10 calories per ounce, that Powerade is almost as bad as a can of Coke, which has 12 per ounce. "Unless you're exercising vigorously, you don't need sports drinks. They have a lot of empty calories, just like anything else," she says.

Most people would agree that their love affair with the sweet stuff—whatever flavor it might be—isn't all that healthy, but no one would put it in the same class as a truly bad habit, such as

Our Changing Habits

Americans used to drink more than twice as much milk as soda; not anymore, according to a study published in the *American Journal of Preventive Medicine*.

In 1978, milk was 8 percent of an American's daily calories. In 2001, it made up just 5 percent.

Soda, on the other hand, was just 3 percent of daily calories in 1978 but 7 percent of daily calories in 2001.

smoking or drinking alcohol to excess, right?

Wrong. Scientists are beginning to do just that. The bulk of the research has focused on connecting the dots between consumption of sugar-sweetened beverages and weight gain, but there is mounting evidence that our national obsession with liquid candy affects more than just our figures. From the very first sip, experts say, cola starts to wreak havoc on the body. It corrodes the teeth, confuses the appetite-regulating hormones in the digestive tract, attacks the bones, and encourages the organ breakdown that leads to diabetes.

Arndt, for one, is convinced that soda was the primary cause of her problems: "I tried to eat somewhat healthy, but my doctors weren't happy about how much I drank, and they attributed my weight in part to that. And going to the dentist was never fun. The dentist would always say, 'Lay off the soda.'" In December 2005, she made the decision to get healthy. With the help of Jenny Craig and Curves, she kicked her soda habit and lost 90 pounds in 7 months.

"I feel incredible," she says.

It's time for us all to follow Arndt's lead. (For healthy soda substitutes, see "How One Family Kicked the Can" on page 80.) The latest research can't be any clearer: When it comes to your health, soda plays a startling number of dangerous roles, starting with . . .

INSULIN GUZZLER

Drinking soda stresses the body's ability to process sugar. Some scientists suspect that the sweet stuff may help explain why the number of Americans with type 2 diabetes has tripled from 6.6 million in 1980 to 20.8 million today.

In a study published in 2004, researchers from Brigham and Women's Hospital in Boston and Harvard Medical School analyzed data from the Nurses' Health Study II, an ongoing trial tracking the health of more than 51,000 women. None of the participants had diabetes at the onset of the study in 1991. Over the following 8 years, 741 women were diagnosed with the disease. Researchers found that women who drank one or more sugary drinks a day gained more weight and were 83 percent more likely to develop type 2 diabetes than those who imbibed less than once a month.

"Anything that promotes weight gain

increases the risk of diabetes," explains David S. Ludwig, MD, PhD, director of the Optimal Weight for Life Program at Children's Hospital Boston, one of the researchers. "But rapidly absorbed carbohydrates like high fructose corn syrup put more strain on insulin-producing cells than other foods." When sugar enters the bloodstream quickly, the pancreas has to secrete large amounts of insulin for the body to process it. Some scientists believe that the unceasing demands that a soda habit places on the pancreas may ultimately leave it unable to keep up with the body's need for insulin. Also, insulin itself becomes less effective at processing sugar; both conditions contribute to the risk of developing diabetes.

Interestingly, women who consumed a lot of fruit juice—which is high in natural fructose—were not at increased risk of diabetes, leading researchers to speculate that naturally occurring sugars may have different metabolic effects than added sugars. They also speculate that vitamins, minerals, fiber, and phytochemicals in fruit juices may have a protective effect against weight gain and diabetes, counterbalancing the adverse effects of sugar.

WAIST WIDENER

Sweetened drinks can pack on the pounds. If, on average, we're drinking 18 ounces of liquid candy daily, we're adding about 225 calories to our diets. Over the course of a month, that's almost 7,000 additional calories, which can easily translate to a 2-pound gain. Over a year, these drinks could be adding 24 pounds to our bottom lines.

That seems to be just what's happening: Over the past 4 decades, our increasing consumption of soda has been matched by our ever-expanding waistlines.

"In my estimation, sugary beverages are one of the two leading environmental causes of obesity, perhaps second only to TV viewing in the magnitude of its effect," says Dr. Ludwig. He and colleagues at the Harvard School of Public Health presented the first strong evidence linking soft drink consumption to childhood obesity back in 2001. They tracked the diets of 548 teens for 19 months and found that kids who drank sugar-sweetened beverages regularly were more likely to be overweight than those who didn't. The researchers also found that the odds of becoming obese

The Diet Dilemma

Almost a third of all carbonated beverages sold in the United States are diet. But are these drinks really any healthier? Not particularly, says Michael Jacobson, PhD, executive director of the Center for Science in the Public Interest. "A can of diet soda doesn't contain 10 teaspoons of sugar, but it has its own problems: caffeine, which is a mildly addictive substance; acids that promote dental erosion; and artificial sweeteners, which raise some small safety questions," he says.

Diet sodas may not even help ward off weight gain. When researchers at the University of Texas Health Science Center examined data from the San Antonio Heart Study, a 25-year look at health habits, study author Sharon Fowler, MPH, an epidemiologist at the center, found that the more diet sodas a person drank, the greater his or her risk of becoming overweight.

An explanation may come via a recent animal study by researchers at Purdue University. They found that artificial sweeteners can interfere with the body's natural ability to regulate calorie intake. This could mean people who consume artificially sweetened items are more likely to overindulge.

Most scientists agree that when it comes to bone health, diet drinks are just as harmful as sugar-sweetened ones. Because diet soda lovers tend to substitute these drinks for milk, they're at higher risk of calcium deficiency.

Sugar-free drinks aren't healthier for your pearly whites either. "There's a myth that diet soda is okay because it's not sugary," says Poonam Jain, BDS, MS, director of community dentistry at Southern Illinois University Edwardsville School of Dental Medicine. Her research revealed that diet drinks were nearly as acidic as regular; thus, they, too, can erode tooth enamel and lead to tooth decay.

The safest bet? Experts recommend that drinkers of artificially sweetened beverages switch to the healthiest diet drink of all: water.

increased 60 percent for each can or glass a day of sugar-sweetened soft drinks.

Dr. Ludwig followed up with an intervention study, published in 2006, examining 103 students from a Cambridge, Massachusetts, high school for 6 months. Half were instructed to drink whatever they liked. The other half were asked to stop drinking sugar-sweetened beverages and were given weekly deliveries of their choice of calorie-free options, including bottled waters, seltzers, and diet sodas. The intervention group lost weight—about 1 pound for each month of the study—while the soda drinkers' weight remained about the same.

Everybody knows that these drinks are high in calories (a 12-ounce can contains about 150 calories; the increasingly popular 20-ounce size packs 250). What people don't realize is that these calories may be particularly effective at making people fat. Perhaps because they pass through the stomach more quickly than food, "liquid calories slip past the body's weight-regulating radar system," says Dr. Ludwig. As a result, people who down sugary drinks don't feel as full as those who consume the same amount of calories in solid food.

This theory was borne out by researchers at Purdue University who, in 2000, gave 15 volunteers 450 calories a day of either soda or jelly beans for a month and then switched them for the next month, while monitoring their total calories. The candy eaters compensated for the extra calories by eating less food and maintained their weight; during the soda phase, the volunteers ate more and gained.

Liquid sugar is a problem, but the type of sugar used in the majority of soft drinks may be making things worse. Although the research is controversial, there's evidence that the high fructose corn syrup used in most sodas fails to suppress the production of ghrelin, a

Liquid Candy

A 2-liter bottle of soda contains the equivalent of 56 cubes of sugar.

hormone made by the stomach that stimulates appetite.

"Unlike carbohydrates containing 100 percent glucose, such as the starch found in rice, potatoes, bread, and pasta, fructose doesn't seem to trigger the hormones that help you regulate appetite and fat storage," says Peter Havel, PhD, a nutrition researcher at the University of California, Davis. "So the body never gets the message to stop eating." Drink a six-pack of cola—900 calories, or about half of the total calories the average woman would need for a day—and your body feels no fuller than if you'd just swallowed water.

TOOTH ROBBER

Sipping on cola is like bathing your mouth in corrosive acid. "Soda eats up and dissolves the tooth enamel," says Poonam Jain, BDS, MS, director of community dentistry at Southern Illinois University Edwardsville School of Dental Medicine.

In a series of studies, Jain tested various sodas by measuring their pH—an indication of acidity. Battery acid, for example, has a pH of 1; water scores a 7. Jain found that sugar-sweetened sodas came in at about 2.5, while diet sodas scored 3.2.

"The acidity can dissolve the mineral content of the enamel, making the teeth weaker, more sensitive, and more susceptible to decay," says Jain. Soda's acidity makes it even worse for teeth than the solid sugar found in candy. By eroding the enamel, soda speeds up the decay process, making it easier for bacteria to enter the teeth.

Savoring soda slowly may damage teeth more than gulping it down, Jain says. "As soon as you take a sip, it acidifies the saliva, which the body then works to neutralize." If you gulp the whole can, the saliva will return to normal in 20 minutes. "But people don't drink soda that way. They take sips over an hour or an hour and a half, and the mouth stays acidic the entire time. This is particularly an issue for people who drink several sodas a day, because they never give their saliva a chance to neutralize," she says.

Several studies, including a University of Michigan analysis of dental checkup data from the Third National Health and Nutrition Examination Survey, confirm that adults who drink three or more sodas a day have up to 62 percent more decayed, missing, and filled teeth than those who drink less.

BONE WRECKER

In the 1950s, children drank 3 cups of milk for every 1 cup of sugary drinks. Today that ratio is reversed: 3 cups of sugary drinks for every cup of milk. Tellingly, osteoporosis is a major health threat for 44 million Americans. Most experts now say that the real culprit is soda's displacement of milk in the diet, though some scientists believe that the acidity of colas may be weakening bones by promoting the loss of calcium.

Whatever the causes of bone loss, the group that stands to suffer the most harm is adolescent girls. In a study of 460 high schoolers in 2000, research at the Harvard School of Public Health found that girls who drank carbonated soft drinks were three times as likely to break their arms and legs as those who consumed other drinks. Dark drinks such as Coca-Cola, Pepsi, and Dr Pepper seemed to be even more dangerous than fruit-flavored sodas such as Sprite: Girls who downed colas were five times as likely to break arms and legs in their teen years as girls who abstained from carbonated beverages. Grace Wyshak, PhD, a biostatistician and the study's lead researcher, believes something in colas is interfering with the body's ability to use calcium. This is a big problem, she says, "because girls will be more susceptible to fractures later in life if they don't acquire optimal bone mass in adolescence."

SODA SOLUTIONS

Diabetes. Obesity. Osteoporosis. Tooth decay. The innocent image of '50s teens sipping soda at the local malt shop is on the wane. And while America seems to be waking up to the corrosive effects of soft drinks—sales dipped 7 percent from 1998 to 2004—it appears sodas are being pushed aside by equally sugary competitors like sports and juice drinks.

Despite lower sales, the soft drink industry insists the studies aren't convincing enough to suggest that soft drinks are contributing to obesity or any other disease. Researchers haven't proven that "one single food or beverage causes obesity," says Richard Adamson, PhD, senior scientific consultant for the American Beverage Association.

How One Family Kicked the Can

Patti Moore confesses that growing up, her family members were the original soda addicts. "The rule at dinner was once you finished your glass of milk, you could have a cola," says Patti, now 45. "I detested milk and would dump it down the bathroom sink, just so I could have my Coke."

Today, a single mother with four daughters in Hamden, Connecticut, Patti has brought the tradition to her own table. Three of her daughters work in fast-food joints with easy access to soda, so she estimates that her family easily downs 2 liters of liquid sugar a day. "Even though none of us have any major weight issues, I know it's not healthy," she says.

She and the girls agreed to a beverage makeover with Christopher Mohr, PhD, RD, owner of Mohr Results, a nutrition and exercise consultation company in Louisville, Kentucky. He suggested the family wean themselves by sprucing up their beverages with these tricks.

Get fizzy. Soda junkies don't just crave sugar. "Carbonation is a big part of the pleasure, too," he says. He advised mixing seltzer with a splash of 100 percent fruit juice or trying one of the new seltzer-juice combos with no added sugar, such as IZZE Sparkling Pomegranate.

Recharge. You can't deny yourself, so go ahead and have caffeine, says Dr. Mohr. He recommended the family brew their own tea and add oranges and lemons

Still, recent efforts to keep sugar-sweetened sodas out of schools signify that some government officials are concerned enough to at least try to make soda less accessible to kids. School districts in New York City, Los Angeles, and Philadelphia have banned soft drinks from schools. And in a historic agreement with health advocates, the Coca-Cola Company, PepsiCo, and Cadbury Schweppes announced in May that they plan to end voluntarily the sale of nearly all sodas in school vending machines and cafeterias by 2010. They promise to instead of sugar for flavor or grab a bottle of Lipton Diet Iced Tea when they're out and about.

Ice up. When no other beverage will do, Dr. Mohr said they could go ahead and have a cola "treat," but fill the glass to the brim with ice first, so there's less room for soda. Another option: Cut the soda with seltzer.

Keep cool. Dr. Mohr advised that they store a pitcher of water in the fridge: "That way, water stays fresh and cool." Having slices of orange, lemon, lime, or cucumber handy will give water a more appealing flavor.

Shake things up. "The girls should have at least 16 ounces of low-fat milk every day," says Dr. Mohr. To make it more enticing, he recommended they make flavored milkshakes in the blender by adding fruit and ice.

After 7 days, Mom has made great strides. "I drink green tea like it's going out of style," Patti says. "I was mixing it with a splash of orange juice, but now I like it straight." Her usual midday hunger has disappeared (resulting in the loss of 1½ pounds), and she feels more energetic. "Before, I was in a rut," she admits. "I would come home and pass out." Now she plans to go hiking with her boyfriend and use the two Pilates DVDs she purchased last year.

Hesitant at first, her kids are now following her lead. "Just the other night, Sammi, who used to drink Coke 24-7, walked to the store and bought a bottle of green tea," says Patti. "I couldn't believe my eyes."

sell only water, unsweetened juice, and milk to elementary and middle schools; juice drinks, sports drinks, and diet sodas will be permitted only in high schools.

Health advocates are pleased by this cascade of initiatives designed to rescue America's increasingly overweight youth, but they fear too little is being done for the rest of us who are still pounding back 18 ounces of the stuff every day.

"We'd like to see more government action, like taxes on soda and other sweetened drinks, and calorie labeling in restaurants so patrons know just how much they're consuming in those super-sized drink containers," says Michael Jacobson, PhD, executive director of the Center for Science in the Public Interest, a consumer advocacy group in Washington, DC, that pressured beverage makers to the bargaining table with the threat of a lawsuit. Dr. Jacobson dreams of a day when you'll pick up a six-pack of soda and each can will have a different cautionary message. One might warn that sweetened drinks can lead to obe-sity. Another might urge consumers to drink water or calorie-free sodas instead of sweetened drinks. A third might alert people to the link between soda consumption and osteoporosis.

But why wait for the government to confirm and legislate what the best nutrition minds already know? Sugared drinks, in their myriad forms, are an unnecessary and potentially detrimental addition to the American diet. And there is no shortage of perfectly healthy alternatives. C'mon, America, it's time to kick the soda habit.

CHAPTER 9

FOOD HEROES OR ZEROES?

The good news, the bad, and—finally—the bottom line on your favorite foods

Before she orders fish at a restaurant, Linda Becker grills the waiter like a detective. "This isn't farmed salmon, is it?" she'll ask. Once she ascertains that it's not—she refuses to eat fish that she believes swim with antibiotics, pesticides, and feces—she practically asks for the salmon's pedigree and personnel file. Then, Becker, a 53-year-old equestrian and mother of one from Frederick, Maryland, will make her menu choice. And in the end, it will probably be the organic chicken. Becker admits that she's a little food phobic, but with good reason. As a breast cancer survivor, she's trying to avoid exposure to environmental chemicals.

The rest of us may not have the same excuse for our picky eating. We're all a little food nutty, and our phobias could be affecting our health.

Blame the headlines. Soy was a wonder food last year; this year it does bubkes for you and may even cause harm. A daily glass of wine protects your heart but ups your breast cancer risk. Some experts say they're seeing more and more people blacklisting foods with bad reputations.

"People are nutritionally traumatized," says Lisa Dorfman, RD, a dietitian and psychotherapist in Miami. "There are just so many red and orange food alerts that you can handle before you go numb. We've had it."

The truth is, some people with special risks do need to be cautious about their intake of "scary" foods such as fish, coffee, eggs, wine, and soy. The rest of us are just depriving ourselves of their significant health benefits—from reducing the odds of cardiovascular disease and cancer to preventing blindness. Here's how to get over it.

FEAR FACTOR: POLLUTION

Fish—or cut bait?

The Good

Scientists and environmentalists agree on this: "You shouldn't give up fish," says Tim Fitzgerald, a researcher with Environmental Defense, which has produced a suitable-for-refrigerator-posting report on seafood (www.oceansalive.org) called "How Many Meals of This Fish Can I Safely Eat per Month?"

The consensus is that fish is the best source of animal protein you can get, and it is relatively low in fat. Many species pack heart-protective omega-3 fats, and those that don't "are still better than eating a cheeseburger," Fitzgerald says. In Harvard's Nurses' Health Study, which has been following more than 80,000 women for nearly 3 decades, those who ate two to four fish meals a week lowered their heart disease risk by 30 percent and stroke risk by 27 percent.

The Bad

Much of the fish on American tables is contaminated with mercury, a neurotoxin that can cause brain damage, and, to a lesser extent, polychlorinated biphenyls (PCBs), industrial pollutants linked to cancer. Children, women in their childbearing years, and those who are pregnant or nursing are considered high risk and need to restrict their intake of high-mercury fish because the heavy metal can interfere with youngsters' brain development.

Studies have found that mercury exposure even before birth can lead to deficits in language, attention, motor skills, and memory in children. Likewise, PCB-laden fish pose a risk to the tiniest bodies: In studies, children who had been exposed in the womb had persistent deficits in both motor skills and short-term memory.

The Bottom Line

If you don't fall into a high-risk category, eating fish twice a week is good for you. But don't eat the same fish twice in 1 week, and restrict highly polluted species you love (such as swordfish) to an occasional meal.

"Having a variety means you're not going to miss any of the important nutrients, but you're not likely to get too much of something that's bad," says Walter Willett, MD, Fredrick John Stare professor of epidemiology and nutrition at Harvard School of Public Health and one of the leaders of the Nurses' Health Study.

If you are at risk, the EPA recommends that you pass up the fish that top its "most contaminated" list: shark, swordfish, tilefish, and king mackerel. Get your two servings a week (up to 12 ounces) by eating low-mercury seafood such as shrimp, canned light tuna, salmon, pollock, and catfish. (Albacore, or white tuna, has more mercury than light tuna, so limit yourself to 6 ounces a week.) For types of PCB-contaminated fish to avoid, check state advisories at http://epa.gov/waterscience/fish/states.htm.

FEAR FACTOR: CHOLESTEROL

Eggs—incredible, but edible?

The Good

There's substantial evidence that for most people, eggs are not only harmless but healthy. "Eggs have good-quality protein with the essential amino acids; choline, which might play a role in preventing memory loss; and lutein and zeaxanthin, carotenoids that protect the eyes against cataracts and macular degeneration," says Maria Luz Fernandez, PhD, a professor of nutritional sciences at the University of Connecticut.

In Dr. Fernandez's study of 45 healthy men and women ages 60 and older, those who ate as many as three eggs a day didn't raise their heart disease risk at all. After a month, 70 percent had little or no change in their cholesterol. About 30 percent saw an increase in cholesterol, but the good cholesterol (HDL) rose in proportion to the bad (LDL). And that's good.

The Bad

The signature happy-face meal of child-hood—two eggs, sunny-side up, and a grin of bacon strips—is now just a memory that makes us nostalgic for the days when we could eat anything and our knees didn't crackle like Rice Krispies. Today, the average American still eats eggs but fewer than five a week. The reason? Cholesterol. One egg yolk packs close to the daily cholesterol limit of 300 milligrams that the American Heart Association (AHA) says we should observe to avoid cardiovascular disease. You can safely have an egg a day as long as you watch your cholesterol intake from other foods (such as shrimp or pastries containing eggs). But the AHA suggests that people with heart disease or significant cardiovascular risk factors limit cholesterol to 200 milligrams a day. (One small egg has 157 milligrams; one medium, 187 milligrams.) You may be genetically predisposed to absorb more cholesterol from food.

The Bottom Line

Follow the AHA's one-a-day guideline—unless you have diabetes. A Harvard study found that men and women with diabetes who ate an egg a day had $1\frac{1}{2}$ to 2 times the risk of developing heart disease as those who ate up to one per week. If you're otherwise healthy, go ahead and order the omelet, which Dr. Fernandez's research suggests might even help your heart. But just to make sure you're staying healthy, schedule a cholesterol test in 2 or 3 months. If the results show you're okay, go for it.

FEAR FACTOR: CANCER

Soy—the has-been?

The Good

Soy's days as a wonder food seem to be over, but don't spit out that edamame just yet. On the positive side, two studies supporting soy were published 2 months after the AHA questioned soy's cholesterol-lowering claims. One found it modestly protective against breast cancer. The other noted a cardiovascular benefit to a specific group: post-menopausal women with low estrogen and suspected heart disease whose blood chemistry made them receptive to plant estrogens from soy.

"Soy is generally very good," agrees Frank Sacks, MD, a professor of cardiovascular disease prevention at Harvard School of Public Health who served on the AHA soy advisory panel. "There are a lot of other reasons to eat tofu and soy burgers: They contain polyunsaturated fats, are a good source of fiber, and have other vitamins. They're a healthy substitute for saturated fats. People just shouldn't expect them to be of any special benefit."

The Bad

Everything that was so right about soy— its ability to curb heart disease, osteoporosis, and hot flashes—seems to be wrong. Last winter, the AHA released a report by a panel of experts saying there was little or no evidence that soy independently lowers the risk of heart disease. Although promoted as a cholesterol reducer, soy only knocks down harmful blood fats by about 3 percent. "If you came to your doctor with a cholesterol level of 250 and you'd lowered it by 3 percent, he'd say, 'Time for a statin,'" concedes Mark Messina, PhD, a soy researcher and consultant for the soy industry. The committee also cast doubt on soy's ability to quench hot flashes and slow bone loss.

The jury isn't in yet on whether soy, which is mildly estrogenic, may fuel estrogen-positive breast cancer. "But if you're on medications like tamoxifen and aromatase inhibitor drugs, you may want to err on the side of caution and stay away from it," says Karen Collins, RD, nutrition consultant for the American Institute for Cancer Research.

The Bottom Line

If you've had breast cancer but aren't taking estrogen-curbing drugs, eat tempeh without fear. But everyone should stick to soy foods and stay far away from processed foods with added isoflavones, the plant hormones in the bean. "It's one thing to eat tofu and another thing entirely to take supplements," says Dr. Sacks. "We don't really know enough about isoflavones and how estrogenic they are, so we're concerned about people getting excessive amounts."

FEAR FACTOR: HEART ATTACK

Coffee—serious perks?

The Good

More than 2 decades of research has failed to find much wrong with drinking caffeinated coffee other than a potential for java jitters. "The major conclusion we've made is that it's remarkably safe," says Dr. Willett. Recent preliminary research suggests that coffee protects against cirrhosis of the liver and even, yes, diabetes. And coffee seems to be the most common source of antioxidants in the American diet. (Coffee is, after all, a bean.) In studies, it has lowered the risk of type 2 diabetes, liver cancer, gallstones, and even breast cancer in the particularly vulnerable: women with the BRCA1 or BRCA2 genes.

There's also evidence that coffee increases alertness, improves athletic performance, and may preserve memory. "One study showed that elderly women who drank coffee over their lifetime tended to have better memory than those who did not," says Michael P. McDonald, PhD, an assistant professor of pharmacology at Vanderbilt University who is an investigator at its Institute for Coffee Studies.

Coffee may even boost your mood. Vanderbilt is launching a study to find out just how much it perks us up.

Caffeine does raise blood pressure. But the Nurses' Health Study and the later NHS II found no connection between coffee drinking and hypertension in a total of more than 155,000 women.

The Bad

You may want to give up coffee if you're pregnant (some equivocal evidence suggests that caffeine may trigger miscarriage), have trouble sleeping (caffeine is a stimulant), or have heartburn or gastroesophageal reflux disease ("Caffeine loosens the valve at the end of the esophagus and can allow for the backwash of stomach acid," explains gastroenterologist David H. Robbins, MD, of Beth Israel Medical Center in New York City).

And there's the latest caffeine jolt: A recent University of Toronto study found that people with a genetic variant that makes caffeine linger in their bodies—an estimated half of the population—were 36 percent more likely to have a heart attack if they drank 2 or 3 cups a day. That figure went up to 64 percent if they had 4 or more. "My wife told me I ruined a lot of people's morning," confesses study author Ahmed El-Sohemy, PhD, Canada research chair in nutrigenomics.

But there's some good news along with the bad. In Dr. El-Sohemy's study, even genetically vulnerable people who had just 1 cup every day weren't at any greater risk of heart attack than those who didn't drink joe.

The Bottom Line

If you love coffee, don't give it up for health reasons, unless you drink so much you register on the Richter scale. Most experts recommend that you limit yourself to 4 cups a day. If you're concerned that you may carry the problematic caffeine gene (there's no test yet), stick to 1 cup. But make sure what you're drinking is really a cup.

"A cup is 8 ounces of drip coffee, regular ground," says Dr. McDonald. "People who go to Starbucks experience the supersize phenomenon: If it only costs you 50 cents more to go from 8 to 16 ounces, you think, 'Why not?' But that's 2 cups."

However, if you have heart disease, drink only filtered coffee and avoid that double shot of espresso or coffee made in a plunge pot. "There is some suggestion that if coffee's not filtered, it can raise cholesterol levels and slightly increase heart disease risk," says Dr. Willett. "Apparently, the cholesterol-raising factors are caught by the filters."

To brew your java safely at home, try the Aerobie AeroPress (see page 95).

FEAR FACTOR: CANCER

Red wine—the tangled vine?

The Good

There's increasing evidence that alcohol—and red wine in particular—may offer generous health benefits for heart and mind. Studies suggest that drinking moderate amounts daily—one or two servings, comprising 5 ounces of wine, 12 ounces of beer, or 1.5 ounces of 80-proof liquor—may lower heart disease risk by as much as 40 percent, possibly by boosting levels of good cholesterol and suppressing clot formation. In the Nurses' Health Study, women who had one drink a day reduced their odds of cognitive decline as they grew older—and their risk was 20 percent lower than the teetotalers in the group.

The Bad

Although early studies hint that a compound called resveratrol in grapes might inhibit tumor growth, alcohol itself has been linked to a variety of cancers, and multiple studies over the past 2 decades have found it may contribute to about 2 percent of all breast cancers diagnosed in the United States. Worse, the risk starts rising at less than half a glass of alcohol a day. Experts also point out that alcoholism has a strong genetic link. "If many of your immediate family members have a drinking problem, it's probably not a good habit to adopt," says Cindy Moore, RD, director of nutrition therapy at the Cleveland Clinic.

The Bottom Line

Most people can have an alcoholic drink a day without fear, experts say. For women who have or are at high risk of breast cancer, however, there's some danger in imbibing.

"Though the relationship between alcohol and breast cancer is real, it's not a powerful one," explains Dr. Willett. "It's not like smoking and lung cancer, where you could have a 2,000-fold increase in risk. At one drink a day, your risk is 10 percent higher than that of someone who doesn't drink. At two drinks a day, it's 20 percent higher. But the good news is that folic acid can mitigate the excess risk." A 400-microgram supplement could allow you to have that glass a day again.

Chapter 10

NUTRITION KICKED UP A NOTCH

Nine ways to chop, sauté, and stir your way to better health

Having diabetes increases your chances for a host of other conditions, such as cancer, and many complications, such a vision problems. The good news is, the foods that you eat can reduce your risk of these problems. The *better* news is, the way you prepare those foods can make them even healthier yet.

Stocked up on leafy greens? Super. Did you know that sautéing them in a bit of olive oil instead of steaming them will help you absorb up to five times as much of the vision-protecting antioxidant beta-carotene? Buying healthy food is just the first step toward a better diet; preparing it correctly can make or break your nutrient bank. Keep reading for even more surprising nutrition-enhancing prep tips.

FIRE UP HEART PROTECTION

Heating lycopene-rich tomatoes instigates a chemical change that makes the heart-healthy nutrient much easier for your body to absorb. Try halving

Roma tomatoes lengthwise; arrange on a baking sheet, drizzle with olive oil, and season with salt and pepper. Broil for 15 to 20 minutes, until they're slightly shriveled. Adding canned crushed tomatoes or tomato paste to recipes works, too. (They were heated during processing.)

MAXIMIZE CANCER PREVENTION

High temperatures destroy alliinase, garlic's most important cancer-fighting and immunity-boosting enzyme. After chopping, let crushed garlic stand for about 10 to 15 minutes before adding it to a sizzling pan. This allows the pungent herb to generate compounds that blunt the damaging effects of heat, report scientists at Pennsylvania State University and the National Cancer Institute. No time to spare? You can always enjoy raw garlic. We love rubbing it on toasted bread and topping it with chopped tomato and onion and a dash of olive oil for a simple bruschetta.

GET 10 TIMES THE IRON

Cooking with tomatoes, apples, or lemons? Heat acidic foods like these in a cast-iron pot or skillet to spike the amount of the energy-boosting iron you absorb by more than 2,000 percent, suggests a Texas Tech University study. "Some iron from the skillet leaches into the food, but the particles are small enough that you won't be able to see or taste them—and it's perfectly safe," says Cynthia Sass, RD, MPH, a spokesperson for the American Dietetic Association.

Bonus tip: You don't have to pull out a pan; coupling certain iron-rich foods with high-acid ones gives a tenfold boost to your iron absorption. "While the iron in red meat is easily absorbed on its own, the type of iron found in beans, grains, and veggies isn't," Sass says. When making a spinach salad, toss in mango slices to increase the iron payoff. Other healthy combos: beans and tomato sauce or cereal and strawberries.

STRENGTHEN EYES AND BONES

Adding avocado, olive oil, nuts, olives, or another healthy fat source to red, green, orange, and yellow fruits and veggies increases the amount of fat-soluble vitamins, such as A, E, and K.

These nutrients boost vision, improve immunity, and protect against stroke and osteoporosis, respectively. "Fat acts as a transporter for them," explains Sass. The same strategy works for carotenoids, the compounds that give tomatoes and carrots their bright hues.

Proof: A recent study from the Ohio State University Comprehensive Cancer Center found that men and women who ate salsa containing chunks of avocado absorbed 4.4 times as much lycopene and 2.6 times as much beta-carotene than those who enjoyed plain salsa.

STOCK UP ON CALCIUM

If you're preparing homemade chicken soup, it's smart to add a hint of lemon juice, vinegar, or tomato to the mix. Pairing a slightly acidic broth with on-the-bone chicken can up the soup's calcium content by 64 percent, according to researchers at Harvard University and Beth Israel Deaconess Medical Center in Boston. (This stock dissolves the bone's calcium more easily than a nonacidic one would.)

Bonus tip: Other research that was referenced in the Harvard/Beth Israel study has shown that slathering spare-ribs with an acidic, vinegar-based barbecue sauce will dramatically increase the calcium content.

GRILL WITHOUT WORRY

The high heat needed to grill meats can create carcinogenic compounds called heterocyclic amines (HCAs), but marinating can help. When researchers at Lawrence Livermore National Laboratory in Livermore, California, soaked chicken breasts in a mixture of brown sugar, olive oil, cider vinegar, garlic, mustard, lemon juice, and salt for 4 hours, they developed up to 99 percent fewer HCAs after 20 minutes of grilling than unmarinated chicken did. Add an extra antioxidant kick with this herb-packed soak: $1/_2$ cup of balsamic vinegar; 2 tablespoons of fresh rosemary; 1 tablespoon each of olive oil, honey, and minced garlic; and $1/_2$ teaspoon of black pepper.

Bonus tip: Instead of marinating hamburgers (too messy), mix in some rosemary. Research has found that it can slash the production of some HCAs by as much as 72 percent.

FIGHT COLDS AND FLU

When you're slicing and dicing fresh produce, cut large pieces. Lots of small portions expose more of the fruit or vegetable to nutrient-leaching oxygen and light. "A larger cut allows you to hold on to more vitamin C, which helps bolster immunity," says Roberta Larson Duyff, RD, author of the *American Dietetic Association Complete Food and Nutrition Guide.* Quarter carrots, potatoes, and tomatoes instead of dicing them; slice melons into crescents rather than cubing.

RETAIN KEY NUTRIENTS

Save yourself some time—and some key nutrients—by not peeling eggplant, apples, potatoes, and other produce before using. "The peel itself is a natural barrier against nutrient loss, and many vitamins and minerals are found in the outer skin or just below it," Duyff says.

Yam skin is loaded with fiber, and zucchini's is full of lutein, which may help prevent age-related macular degeneration, for example. (Remove grit and pathogens with cold running water and a vegetable brush.)

Bonus tip: Add citrus zest to your favorite recipes. A University of Arizona study linked eating limonene—a compound in lemon, lime, and orange peel—to a 34 percent reduction in skin cancer.

DOUBLE THE ANTIOXIDANTS

Dressing your salad with herbs can more than double its cancer-fighting punch, according to a recent Italian study. When compared with garden salads made with no added herbs, those featuring lemon balm and marjoram had up to 200 percent more antioxidants per serving. Spices such as ginger and cumin also upped the antioxidant quotient.

MEDICAL BREAKTHROUGHS

What's the latest food news? Read on!

TAKE A COFFEE BREAK

A study from the University of Minnesota found that regular coffee drinkers may be less likely to develop diabetes.

Researchers analyzed data gathered from 1986 to 1997 on more than 28,000 postmenopausal women and found that those who had consumed 4 to 6 cups of regular or decaf a day (equivalent to 2 or 3 large cups by today's standards) throughout much of their lives had at least a 22 percent lower risk of the disease than women who abstained.

The experts suspect that compounds and minerals in coffee beans may improve the sensitivity of insulin receptors and help the body process blood sugar more efficiently.

But how you drink your coffee matters a great deal. French presses produce a richer-flavored coffee than regular drip-brewed but allow chemicals to slip through that research shows boost "bad" LDL cholesterol levels by 10 percent. The Aerobie AeroPress, for example, uses filters to cull those compounds and distill delicious coffee without the bitterness produced by other French presses. (They're sold at independent coffee shops. See the complete list at www.aerobie.com).

If caffeine makes you more jittery than a jitterbug, it just got a lot easier to figure out how much caffeine you really drink. (Hint: Your morning coffee is just the beginning.) One stealthy source: soda. Both Pepsi and Coca-Cola recently began disclosing the amount of caffeine in each 8-ounce serving (up to 50 milligrams). That's not necessarily bad, as long as you cap your total daily caffeine intake at 200 to 300 milligrams (or 2 to 3 cups of coffee); research suggests that this amount is safe, boosts your alertness, and may even reduce your risk of Alzheimer's disease. However, if you go overboard or show signs of caffeine sensitivity—such as headaches, anxiety, or gastrointestinal distress—or are taking certain antibiotics or antianxiety meds, cutting back on soda or coffee (your choice!) may be a wise move.

TAKE D TO PROTECT AGAINST THE BIG D

Getting adequate vitamin D daily in food and supplements may help stop type 2 diabetes, say Tufts University researchers. In their 20-year study of 81,700 women, those with the highest vitamin D intake had a 28 percent lower risk of type 2 diabetes than those with the lowest. Good food sources: milk, fatty fish, and eggs.

SCREAM FOR ICE CREAM

Can ice cream fight diabetes? Just maybe. First it fought fat. Now comes evidence that eating low-fat dairy foods may reduce your risk of developing type 2 diabetes. When Harvard University researchers monitored the diets of more than 41,000 men for 12 years, they discovered that for every daily serving of low-fat dairy eaten, a man's risk of developing diabetes dropped by 9 percent.

Calcium and other nutrients may play roles, says study author Hyon Choi, MD, DPH, although Dr. Choi found that people who eat more low-fat dairy tend to have healthier diets overall.

The biggest surprise: In addition to yogurt, fat-free milk, and the other usual suspects, this study also included low-fat ice cream. Our favorite brand: Edy's Slow Churned Rich & Creamy Light, which has half the saturated fat of regular but all the flavor.

SPICE IT UP

While apple pie and other goodies might be less than helpful for diabetes, the spice that flavors them might be just the opposite. Researchers are finding that cinnamon extract can help lower blood sugar.

Cinnamomum cassia is the dried bark of evergreen trees cultivated throughout Asia. As early as 2700 BC, Chinese herbalists treated diarrhea and kidney disorders with cinnamon. Later, Greek healers and practitioners of Indian Ayurvedic medicine valued it as a remedy for digestive problems.

Cinnamon may help lower cholesterol and triglycerides. Pakistani researchers gave 60 type 2 diabetics with borderline-high lipid levels a daily placebo pill or one with 1 to 6 grams of cinnamon. After 40 days, those in the cinnamon group saw their cholesterol levels fall by at least 13 percent and their triglyceride levels by at least 23 percent. The placebo had no effect.

Newer research shows that cinnamon can help rein in blood sugar. German researchers collected blood from 65 adults with type 2 diabetes who then took a capsule containing the equivalent of 1 gram of cinnamon powder or a placebo three times a day for 4 months. By the end, cinnamon reduced blood sugar by about 10 percent; the placebo users improved by only 4 percent. Compounds in cinnamon may activate enzymes that stimulate insulin receptors.

The extract used in the study is sold only in Europe, but Envita Labs' Cinna-BeticII is similar. (Stick with the extract, which is water soluble; large amounts of the actual spice can be dangerous.) It's available at vitamin retailers. Follow label instructions.

EAT FOR YOUR GENES

African Americans, Asians, and Hispanics can reduce their risk of developing diabetes by a whopping 46 percent just by making some easy changes in their eating habits, according to Harvard researchers who followed more than 78,000 women for 20 years. That's a big health payoff: These groups tend to have a much higher risk of the disease than Caucasians (who get only a 23 percent reduction in risk by munching wisely).

One of the most crucial shifts: favoring low-glycemic foods—which studies show help stabilize your blood sugar. Try these simple strategies.

• Swap sugary drinks, such as soda and bottled sweetened teas, for water and freshly brewed unsweetened teas.
• Ditch refined grains, such as white rice, for fiber-rich whole grains, such as brown rice or quinoa.
• Pass on foods that contain saturated fats or trans fats; instead, pick foods rich in polyunsaturated fats, including fish and nuts.

• Keep meat choices lean, and incorporate other sources of protein into your diet, too. Try chickpeas and kidney and black beans.

CRUSH DIABETES WITH CARROTS

Their brilliant orange color means they're bursting with carotenoids, antioxidants that may help prevent diabetes, suggests new research from the University of Minnesota School of Public Health. Among 4,500 people tested over 15 years, those with the highest levels of carotenoids in their blood had about half the diabetes risk of those with the least.

Try the Sweet 'n' Tangy Carrots recipe (see page 303), which makes four half-cup servings. Snack on them over the next 7 days and you'll meet your carotenoid goal for the week.

EAT MORE FIBER

According to researchers at the German Institute of Human Nutrition in Potsdam-Rehbrücke, 17 overweight or obese people who ate 31 grams of insoluble fiber every day experienced an 8 percent jump in insulin sensitivity. That's the amount of fiber in three servings of high-fiber cereal or two servings of barley.

BE A LITTLE SEEDY

Eating more magnesium can reduce your risk of type 2 diabetes. Tufts University scientists found that adults consuming the most magnesium—more than 386 milligrams daily—were less likely to have insulin resistance than those downing the least.

"Insulin resistance means your cells don't respond well to insulin, a hormone that moves sugar out of your blood," says study author Nicola M. McKeown, PhD.

Boost your magnesium intake with sunflower seeds; each ounce contains 37 milligrams of the mineral.

Success Story
She Trans-Formed Her Diet

Until recently, trans fats fell into a broad category of things that Amy O'Connor, former deputy editor for *Prevention*, knew weren't healthy but ate anyway because, well, she's busy paying bills and trying to keep her toddler from flinging the cat off the terrace. Besides, how much damage could a little artificial fat do?

Plenty, according to Jeffrey Aron, MD, an assistant clinical professor of medicine at the University of California, San Francisco. "Emerging data strongly suggests that cancer and dementia are made worse by trans fats," he told her. "Putting trans fats into your body is like dropping fine grains of sand into a Swiss watch. Eventually, the system shuts down." Yikes. Even if your body runs more like a Timex than a Rolex, you still want to keep it ticking for as long as possible.

Ironically, nutritionists used to think trans fats were the healthy alternative to saturated fat, but that was before the evidence against them started piling up. In the 1990s, at least six major studies found that trans fats raised the ratio of "bad" LDL cholesterol to "good" HDL cholesterol; other research has found that trans fats can raise triglycerides, another risk factor for heart disease. Three large investigations—the Health Professionals Follow-Up Study; the Nurses' Health Study; and the Alpha-Tocopherol, Beta-Carotene Cancer Prevention Trial— strengthened the link between heart attacks and trans fats. Researchers suggest a reason: Trans fats trigger widespread systemic inflammation.

Currently, the USDA advises that we simply watch our intake (average daily consumption is about 5.8 grams). But the accumulating anti-trans research has led some public health groups to suggest tighter limits. The American Heart Association, for one, recommends reducing your intake to less than 1 percent of daily calories, or about 2 grams. And the Center for Science in the Public Interest (CPSI), a Washington, DC, nutrition-policy advocacy group, urges a zero-tolerance

(continued)

Success Story (cont.)

policy. As CSPI head Michael F. Jacobson, PhD, explains, "Trans fats account for as many as 50,000 deaths a year." When Amy heard that, she vowed to ban them from her household.

Unfortunately, that wasn't as easy as she'd originally hoped, because trans fats are found almost everywhere a busy mom might look. They're usually created when vegetable oil is hydrogenated—altered with hydrogen—to make it solid at room temperature (think oil versus margarine). That solidity helps make potato chips crunchy and piecrusts tender. It also makes food more shelf stable, which means if a food is boxed or wrapped and sold in a grocery store, there's a good chance trans fats are lurking inside. So Amy called in the nutrition experts to help her navigate three square meals. Here are the lessons she learned along the way to trans-freedom.

Lesson 1: Labels Don't Tell You Everything

Since last January, federal law has mandated that all Nutrition Facts labels list trans fats under the line item for saturated fat. Simply by checking labels at the supermarket, Amy discovered that Oreo cookies and other favorite treats are now trans free. Triscuits, Wheat Thins, Chips Ahoy, Mallomars, Boca products, Honey Maid low-fat cinnamon grahams, and some SnackWell's cookies also contain zero trans fat.

But when Amy checked in with Dr. Jacobson, he wasn't impressed. That's because some of the foods labeled 'trans-fat free' aren't. "That packaging can be deceptive," he says. "When it says 'zero gram trans fat,' by law it can contain up to half a gram per serving." A few servings a day, and you could find yourself in dangerous trans-land.

Still, it is possible to shop smart. Stores like Whole Foods and Wild Oats Markets have instituted a total ban. Otherwise, scrutinize the ingredients list; the words *hydrogenated* or *partially hydrogenated* are the number one tip-off that trans fats are present. Finally, search out USDA-certified organic products; the process of hydrogenation is forbidden under current organics regulations.

Lesson 2: Even Healthy Foods Have Some Trans

Pizza, pancakes, and potpie form the pyramid that is O'Connor's 18-month-old's diet. She found trans fats in every one. She replaced the pies and pancake mix with trans-free alternatives—Amy's brand Country Vegetable Pie and Bisquick Heart Smart—and swapped the frozen pizzas with safer picks from Healthy Choice.

Then Dr. Aron and Dr. Jacobson told Amy that negligible amounts of trans fats occur naturally in meat and milk. The catch: Her husband will move out if she makes him become a vegan. Since these tiny levels pose no harm, according to experts, the family plans to live with natural trans.

Lesson 3: Menus Are Minefields

There's no law that says restaurants, delis, or coffee shops have to reveal their ingredients, so finding the trans fats on a menu is nearly impossible. But they're there; restaurants generally use them because they're more stable than other cooking oils. Many popular chains, including Au Bon Pain, Panera Bread, California Pizza Kitchen, and Wendy's, to their credit, have switched to healthier oils; those that haven't offer complete nutritional information online. (That's where Amy learned that her favorite Starbucks pumpkin scone weighs in at a whopping 6 grams of trans fats. Thankfully, the equally tasty raspberry scone is trans free.) To further protect diners, some local governments, such as in New York City, have moved to institute bans.

One night, when placing a take-out order, Amy was thrilled to hear that the local barbecue joint has jumped on the no-trans bandwagon. The feast arrives, and she settles in with a big ol' plate of coleslaw, tangy baked beans, and delightfully greasy short ribs. No trans—but lots of finger-lickin' saturated fat. Oh well, that's another story.

PART III

LOSE WEIGHT

CHAPTER 11

28 DAYS TO A NEW YOU

Get slim, strong, and powerful with fat-blasting cardio, firm-all-over moves, and an energy-boosting eating plan

Yes, you have great intentions. But juggling work, family, and home leaves you little time for that last item on your to-do list: you—and getting into a shape you're happy about. No worries; it's not too late. With our new plan, you can still shed up to 10 pounds, firm and tone, and lose inches—all in just a month! Keep going, and you'll lose even more—at the rate of about 1 to 2 pounds a week.

Studies have confirmed that when it comes to weight loss, programs that combine diet and exercise are superior to dieting alone because they preserve muscle—the key to keeping your metabolism in high gear. And that's the basis of this full-body shape-up plan. We help you maximize your efforts with progressive calorie-burning cardio workouts and strength moves that target multiple muscles at the same time. The balanced diet is portion- and calorie-controlled, so it's almost impossible to slip up.

A plus: The meals are packed with fat-fighting fiber, which keeps you satisfied, boosts your energy, and helps you lose more weight. A University of Rhode Island study found that women who combined exercise with a high-fiber, low-calorie diet similar to ours lost three times as much weight over 24 weeks as those who exercised without changing their eating habits. Plus, you'll start seeing results in as little as 2 weeks, which is great incentive to keep you on track.

Sure, the program is intense (though we do give you a few rest days!), but we'll be with you every step of the way. (Nina Moore, a certified trainer at the Sports Club/LA who's worked with clients for more than 13 years, designed this plan.) And just think of the payoff:

You'll be at least a size smaller in just 28 days!

THE WORKOUT

Trim down with calorie-burning cardio routines, and tone up with metabolism-revving strength moves (pages 116 to 123).

At a Glance

Three days a week: Do Fat-Blasting Cardio (see "The Plan," opposite). Alternate between progressively fast and slow intervals of the activity of your choice. This doubles your weight loss without doubling your workout time.

Two days a week: Strength-train (see page 116). Tone up with sculpting exercises that hit multiple muscle groups at

---

Your Cardio Intensity

Use this 1-to-10 scale to maximize your calorie burn during Fat-Blasting Cardio.

Warm-up, cool-down (3–4 intensity level): easy enough that you can sing

Slow pace (5–6 intensity level): moderate enough that you can talk freely

Quick pace (7–8 intensity level): brisk enough that you can talk, but you'd rather not the same time, so you get a full workout in only four moves.

One day a week: Cross-train. Pick a fun cardio activity to keep your calorie burn and motivation high and your risk of injury low.

What you'll need: a chair or bench, an exercise mat, and sets of 3- and 5-pound dumbbells. The weight should be hard to lift by the end of each set. If it's still fairly effortless for you, increase the weight.

The Plan

Day 1: Fat-Blasting Cardio: 28 minutes

5-minute warmup (3–4 intensity level, progressing to 5–6 by minute 4)

2-minute fast walk* at a quick pace (7–8 intensity level)

1-minute slow walk (5–6 intensity level)

Repeat fast/slow sequence 6 times.

5-minute cooldown (3–4 intensity level)

Day 2: Strength-Train A: Core Control (see page 116.)

Do 2 sets of 10 to 12 reps of each exercise, resting 1 minute between sets.

Day 3: Fat-Blasting Cardio: 34 minutes

5-minute warmup (3–4 intensity level, progressing to 5–6 by minute 4)

3-minute fast walk at a quick pace (7–8 intensity level)

1-minute slow walk (5–6 intensity level)

Repeat fast/slow sequence 6 times.

5-minute cooldown (3–4 intensity level)

Day 4: Strength-Train B: Butt Camp (see page 120.)

Do 2 sets of 10 to 12 reps of each exercise, resting 1 minute between sets.

Day 5: Repeat Day 3.

Day 6: Cross-train for 30 minutes.

Give your cardio a kick by doing something new: inline skating (burns 816 calories per hour), bicycling (544 per hour), or dancing (442 per hour**).

Day 7: Rest.

Day 8: Fat-Blasting Cardio: 40 minutes

5-minute warmup (3–4 intensity level, progressing to 5–6 by minute 4)

5-minute fast walk at a quick pace (7–8 intensity level)

1-minute slow walk (5–6 intensity level)

Repeat fast/slow sequence 5 times.

5-minute cooldown (3–4 intensity level)

Day 9: Strength-Train A: Core Control

Do 3 sets of 10 to 12 reps of each exercise, resting 1 minute between sets; up the amount of weight you lift on the first set, and on the second set if possible.

---

*You may substitute swimming, jogging, cycling, etc. for walking.

**All calculations are based on a 150-pound woman.

Day 10: Fat-Blasting Cardio: 45 minutes

5-minute warmup (3–4 intensity level, progressing to 5–6 by minute 4)

6-minute fast walk at a quick pace (7–8 intensity level)

1-minute slow walk (5–6 intensity level)

Repeat fast/slow sequence 5 times.

5-minute cooldown (3–4 intensity level)

Day 11: Strength-Train B: Butt Camp

Do 3 sets of 10 to 12 reps of each exercise, resting 1 minute between sets; up the amount of weight you lift on the first set if possible.

Day 12: Repeat Day 10.

Day 13: Cross-train for 40 minutes.

Beat boredom. Try an activity or class you've never done before—kickboxing (burns 680 calories per hour) or Power Yoga (burns about 306 per hour).

Day 14: Rest.

Day 15: Fat-Blasting Cardio: 43 minutes

5-minute warmup (3–4 intensity level, progressing to 5–6 by minute 4)

10-minute fast walk at a quick pace (7–8 intensity level)

1-minute slow walk (5–6 intensity level)

Repeat fast/slow sequence 3 times.

5-minute cooldown (3–4 intensity level)

Day 16: Strength: Core Control

Try the "make it harder" moves or increase weight lifted. Do 2 sets of 10 to 12 reps of each exercise, resting 45 seconds between sets.

Day 17: Fat-Blasting Cardio: 42 minutes

5-minute warmup (3–4 intensity level, progressing to 5–6 by minute 4)

15-minute fast walk at a quick pace (7–8 intensity level)

1-minute slow walk (5–6 intensity level)

Repeat fast/slow sequence 2 times.

5-minute cooldown (3–4 intensity level)

Day 18: Strength-Train B: Butt Camp

Try the "make it harder" moves or increase weight lifted. Do 2 sets of 10 to 12 reps of each exercise, resting 45 seconds between sets.

Day 19: Repeat Day 17.

Day 20: Cross-train for 50 minutes.

Anybody for swimming (burns up to 680 calories an hour)? Just be sure to keep your heart rate up during the cardio of your choice.

Day 21: Rest.

Day 22: Fat-Blasting Cardio: 45 minutes

5-minute warmup (3–4 intensity level, progressing to 5–6 by minute 4)

35-minute fast walk at a quick pace (7–8 intensity level)

5-minute cooldown (3–4 intensity level)

Day 23: Strength-Train A: Core Control

Do 3 sets of 10 to 12 reps of each exercise (do the "make it harder" version whenever possible), resting 30 seconds between sets.

Day 24: Fat-Blasting Cardio: 50 minutes

5-minute warmup (3–4 intensity level, progressing to 5–6 by minute 4)

40-minute fast walk at a quick pace (7–8 intensity level)

5-minute cooldown (3–4 intensity level)

Day 25: Strength-Train B: Butt Camp

Do 3 sets of 10 to 12 reps of each exercise (do the "make it harder" version whenever possible), resting 30 seconds between sets.

Day 26: Repeat Day 24.

Day 27: Cross-train for 60 minutes.

Hiking, biking, inline skating, basketball, tennis, racquetball, or a combination—it's up to you. The only requirement is that you keep your heart rate up for an hour.

Day 28: Beach day!

THE DIET

Mix and match these low-cal, easy, energizing options to create your own perfect meal plan that'll slim you down.

At a Glance

Each day, you choose one easy-to-prepare breakfast, lunch, dinner, and snack that together deliver a total of 1,800 calories and 25 grams of fat-fighting fiber (we did the counting for you).

The Plan

What's not to love about our easy-to-follow regimen? Every meal contains a fat-fighting dose of fiber (an average of 25 grams a day), the nutrient that slims you down by filling you up. A recent University of Minnesota study found that people who ate the most vegetables, fruits, and other fiber-rich foods lost 2 to 3 pounds more per month than those on lower-fiber diets—and that can add up to a whopping 30 pounds in a year. The meals are also loaded with bone-building calcium (about 1,200 milligrams a day), which has been found to kick-start the body's fat-burning engines.

Here's how the plan works: Each day, choose a breakfast (400 calories each), lunch (550 calories), dinner (650 calories), and snack (200 calories). To keep the recipes diabetes-friendly, each meal has less than 75 grams of carbohydrate. We've even taken into account that you don't always have time to cook (try a frozen entrée option). Combine the plan with our exercise plan, and then break out the skinny jeans: Your new body will be ready for them!

Take Your Pick:
Breakfast (400 calories)

The 5-Minute Breakfast: Toast 1 slice 100% whole wheat raisin bread and spread with 1 tablespoon peanut butter. Serve with 1 cup low-fat plain yogurt and 1 cup strawberries, sliced.

398 cal, 20 g pro, 50 g carb, 13.5 g fat, 4.5 g sat fat, 15 mg chol, 8 g fiber, 437 mg sodium, 500 mg calcium

Diet Exchanges: 2 milk, 0 vegetable, 1 fruit, 1 starch/bread, 1 meat, 1.5 fat

Homemade Muesli: Mix $^1/_2$ cup uncooked rolled oats; 1 medium tart apple, chopped; and 1 tablespoon slivered almonds. Top with $^2/_3$ cup light soy milk or fat-free milk. Serve with 6 ounces calcium- and vitamin D–fortified orange juice.

431 cal, 15 g pro, 80 g carb, 7 g fat, 0.5 g sat fat, 0 mg chol, 11 g fiber, 73 mg sodium, 456 mg calcium

Diet Exchanges: 1 milk, 0 vegetable, 2.5 fruit, 2 starch/bread, 0.5 meat, 1 fat

Breakfast Burrito: In nonstick pan, scramble 1 whole egg and 1 egg white (or $^1/_2$ cup liquid egg substitute). Fill a warmed 10$^1/_2$" whole wheat tortilla with cooked egg, 1 ounce shredded low-fat Cheddar cheese, 2 tablespoons salsa, 3 tablespoons chopped tomato, and 3 tablespoons chopped cilantro. Serve with 1 cup cubed melon (such as honeydew or cantaloupe).

347 cal, 21 g pro, 36 g carb, 14 g fat, 5 g sat fat, 232 mg chol, 5 g fiber, 731 mg sodium, 454 mg calcium

Diet Exchanges: 0 milk, 1 vegetable, 1 fruit, 0 starch/bread, 2 meat, 1 fat

Latte & Muffin: Mix $^2/_3$ cup warm 1% milk with strong coffee. Top a 2-ounce (Ping-Pong ball–size) mini bran muffin with 1 tablespoon peanut butter and serve with fruit salad ($^1/_2$ medium orange, peeled and chopped, and 1 kiwifruit, peeled and chopped).

401 cal, 14 g pro, 65 g carb, 16 g fat, 3 g sat fat, 8 mg chol, 7 g fiber, 415 mg sodium, 293 mg calcium

Diet Exchanges: 1 milk, 0 vegetable, 1.5 fruit, 3 starch/bread, 1 meat, 1.5 fat

Berry Ricotta Toast: Top 1 slice 100% whole wheat toast with 1 tablespoon jam and $^1/_3$ cup part-skim ricotta. Serve with $^2/_3$ cup blueberries, 6 ounces grapefruit juice, and 1 cup coffee with $^1/_3$ cup 1% milk.

402 cal, 16 g pro, 64 g carb, 9 g fat, 5 g sat fat, 28 mg chol, 5 g fiber, 328 mg sodium, 373 mg calcium

Diet Exchanges: 0.5 milk, 0 vegetable, 2 fruit, 1.5 starch/bread, 1.5 meat, 1 fat

Orange Sunshine Pancakes: In medium bowl, combine $^1/_2$ cup 1% milk; $^1/_3$ cup low-fat, low-sodium pancake mix; 2 tablespoons liquid egg substitute; 4 teaspoons toasted wheat germ; 1 tablespoon orange juice concentrate; and 1 teaspoon grated orange zest. Pour 2 circles of batter onto hot griddle coated with cooking spray and cook until bubbles begin to pop. Flip and cook 2 minutes or until done. Top with 2 tablespoons marmalade and $^1/_3$ cup fat-free plain yogurt.

400 cal, 17 g pro, 75 g carb, 6 g fat, 1.5 g sat fat, 4 mg chol, 2 g fiber, 171 mg sodium, 340 mg calcium

Diet Exchanges: 1 milk, 0 vegetable, 0.5 fruit, 2 starch/bread, 3 meat, 0.5 fat

Vegetable Omelet: In small pan coated with cooking spray, sauté 2 tablespoons each diced onion and green bell pepper until tender, approximately 3 minutes. Remove. In same pan, add $^3/_4$ cup liquid egg substitute and cook over low heat until firm. Add onion-pepper mixture and $^1/_2$ cup diced tomato, then fold egg in half. Serve with 1 slice 100% whole wheat toast topped with 2 teaspoons jam and 8 ounces calcium- and vitamin D–fortified orange juice.

396 cal, 28 g pro, 53 g carb, 8 g fat, 2 g sat fat, 2 mg chol, 4 g fiber, 514 mg sodium, 408 mg calcium

Diet Exchanges: 0 milk, 1 vegetable, 1.5 fruit, 1 starch/bread, 3 meat, 1 fat

Fruity Parfait: In tall glass, layer $^1/_3$ cup low-fat granola; 1 cup low-fat plain yogurt; 1 medium orange, peeled and chopped; 1 kiwifruit, peeled and chopped; and 2 teaspoons dried fruit (apricots, raisins, etc.).

403 cal, 18 g pro, 71 g carb, 6 g fat, 2.5 g sat fat, 15 mg chol, 8 g fiber, 237 mg sodium, 522 mg calcium

Diet Exchanges: 2 milk, 0 vegetable, 2 fruit, 1 starch/bread, 0 meat, 0 fat

Take Your Pick:
Lunch (550 calories)

Make-Your-Own Salad: Top 4 cups chopped romaine lettuce with 1 ounce shredded low-fat Cheddar cheese; $^1/_3$ cup corn; $^1/_3$ cup canned beans (such as black or kidney), rinsed and drained; 2 tablespoons grated carrots; 4 tablespoons diced red onion; 4 ounces roasted or grilled chicken breast (about the size of your palm); 2 tablespoons balsamic vinegar; and dash of extra-virgin olive oil (less than 1 teaspoon). Serve with 1 medium whole wheat roll spread with 1 teaspoon butter.

554 cal, 53 g pro, 53 g carb, 17 g fat, 6 g sat fat, 112 mg chol, 14 g fiber, 471 mg sodium, 371 mg calcium

Diet Exchanges: 0 milk, 4 vegetable, 0 fruit, 2 starch/bread, 6 meat, 2 fat

Gazpacho and Grilled Cheese: Gazpacho: In blender, puree 2 cups peeled and chopped tomatoes; $^1/_2$ green bell pepper, chopped; $^1/_3$ cup chopped onion; 1 clove garlic; $^1/_3$ cup chopped peeled cucumber; 1 tablespoon balsamic vinegar; 2 teaspoons olive oil; and salt and black pepper to taste. (Strain for smoother texture.) Grilled Cheese: Spread 1 teaspoon Dijon mustard on 2 slices low-carb 100% whole wheat bread. Add $1^1/_2$ ounce low-fat Cheddar cheese, sliced, and $^1/_2$ cup bottled roasted red peppers, drained. In nonstick pan, grill on each side until cheese is melted. Serve with 1 cup sparkling water mixed with $^1/_3$ cup calcium- and vitamin D–fortified orange juice over crushed ice.

491 cal, 24 g pro, 57 g carb, 22 g fat, 7 g sat fat, 30 mg chol, 13 g fiber, 418 mg sodium, 858 mg calcium

Diet Exchanges: 0 milk, 4 vegetable, 0.5 fruit, 1.5 starch/bread, 1.5 meat, 3 fat

Mango Chicken Sandwich: Spread 1 tablespoon hoisin sauce on 2 slices sourdough bread (70 calories per slice).

Add 3 ounces roasted or grilled chicken breast; $^1/_4$ fresh mango, peeled and sliced; 1 slice red onion; and 2 tablespoons chopped cilantro. Serve with Spinach-Orange Salad: Toss 3 cups bagged baby spinach leaves with $^1/_2$ cup canned mandarin orange slices, drained; 2 tablespoons diced red onion; and 1 tablespoon dried cranberries. Dress with 2 tablespoons balsamic vinegar and dash of extra-virgin olive oil (less than 1 teaspoon).

488 cal, 36 g pro, 73 g carb, 7 g fat, 1.5 g sat fat, 73 mg chol, 8 g fiber, 755 mg sodium, 124 mg calcium

Diet Exchanges: 0 milk, 2 vegetable, 1.5 fruit, 2.5 starch/bread, 4 meat, 1 fat

Roast Beef Sandwich: Spread 2 slices 100% whole wheat bread with 1 tablespoon low-fat, low-sodium mayonnaise. Top with 2 thin slices roast beef (about 2 ounces) and 3 lettuce leaves. Serve with 12 baby carrots and 1 medium apple.

353 cal, 19 g pro, 60 g carb, 5.5 g fat, 1 g sat fat, 32 mg chol, 11 g fiber, 770 mg sodium, 55 mg calcium

Diet Exchanges: 0 milk, 2 vegetable, 1 fruit, 2 starch/bread, 2 meat, 0.5 fat

Beef Fajita: In nonstick pan coated with cooking spray, sauté 3 ounces lean sirloin steak strips (prepackaged or cut at home) with $1^1/_4$ cups fresh or frozen red and green bell pepper slices and $^1/_2$ cup onion slices. Stir frequently until strips are cooked through and vegetables are tender (approximately 10 minutes). Toss steak strips and vegetables with 1 tablespoon bottled fajita sauce until well coated. Wrap in a warmed $10^1/_2$" whole wheat tortilla. (Time-saver: You can make these fajitas ahead, wrap individually in microwave-friendly plastic wrap, and reheat in microwave.) For on the side, toss 1 large tomato, diced; $^1/_3$ cup fresh or frozen corn (rinsed and drained); $^1/_4$ cup chopped cilantro or parsley; 3 tablespoons diced red onion; 2 teaspoons balsamic vinegar; and 1 teaspoon extra-virgin olive oil.

428 cal, 26 g pro, 56 g carb, 12 g fat, 2 g sat fat, 40 mg chol, 10 g fiber, 408 mg sodium, 90 mg calcium

Diet Exchanges: 0 milk, 4 vegetable, 0 fruit, 1 starch/bread, 1 meat, 1 fat

Take Your Pick:
Dinner (650 calories)

Cheesy Spinach Pizza: Top one 10" thin pizza crust with 1 cup low-sodium marinara sauce; 6 ounces baby spinach (steamed and drained); 2 cloves garlic,

minced; and 4 ounces shredded low-fat mozzarella cheese. Bake at 400°F until cheese bubbles and pizza is heated through. For on the side, drizzle 2 tablespoons low-fat, low-sodium Italian vinaigrette on 12 inner romaine leaves. Top with 1 tablespoon Parmesan cheese. Serve with 1 cup fresh or frozen and thawed strawberries.

Per 2 slices: 358 cal, 17 g pro, 50 g carb, 11 g fat, 4 g sat fat, 19 mg chol, 6 g fiber, 791 mg sodium, 294 mg calcium

Diet Exchanges: 0 milk, 1 vegetable, 0 fruit, 0.5 starch/bread, 1 meat, 1 fat

Salmon Supper: Drizzle lemon juice on a 5-ounce salmon fillet and broil or grill about 5 minutes per side or until just opaque. Top with $^1/_2$ cup diced mango mixed with $^1/_3$ cup salsa. For on the side, steam $^2/_3$ cup each snow peas and sliced carrots. Serve with 1 cup cooked instant brown rice topped with 1 tablespoon chopped walnuts.

593 cal, 35 g pro, 66 g carb, 22 g fat, 4 g sat fat, 83 mg chol, 7 g fiber, 741 mg sodium, 84 mg calcium

Diet Exchanges: 0 milk, 2 vegetable, 0 fruit, 3 starch/bread, 4 meat, 2 fat

Guiltless Fried Chicken: Smear a 4-ounce skinless, boneless chicken breast with 1 tablespoon trans free margarine and roll in 2 tablespoons dried bread crumbs seasoned with a pinch each of dried thyme and rosemary. Place on baking sheet coated with cooking spray, and bake at 400°F for 35 to 50 minutes, or until center of chicken is no longer pink. Sauté 2 cups asparagus spears and 2 cloves garlic, minced, in 1 teaspoon olive oil. Microwave 6 ounces sweet potato until soft and mash with 2 tablespoons 1% milk and 1 tablespoon chopped pecans.

557 cal, 40 g pro, 58 g carb, 18.5 g fat, 4.4 g sat fat, 67 mg chol, 10 g fiber, 656 mg sodium, 150 mg calcium

Diet Exchanges: 0 milk, 2 vegetable, 0 fruit, 2.5 starch/bread, 4 meat, 3 fat

Pork Tenderloin: Season 4 ounces pork tenderloin with dried herb mix such as rosemary and thyme. Broil or grill until cooked through. Serve with $^2/_3$ cup cooked instant brown rice, $^2/_3$ cup steamed (or microwaved frozen) green peas, and 1 steamed artichoke with 2 tablespoons low-calorie, low-sodium mayonnaise seasoned with black pepper or curry powder.

474 cal, 36 g pro, 62 g carb, 8 g fat, 1.6 g sat fat, 73 mg chol, 13 g fiber, 350 mg sodium, 94 mg calcium

Diet Exchanges: 0 milk, 2.5 vegetable, 0 fruit, 3 starch/bread, 3.5 meat, 1 fat

Steak and Potatoes: Broil or grill 4 ounces lean steak 2 to $2^1/_2$ minutes on each side for rare or 4 to 5 minutes per side if you prefer well done. Serve with 6 ounces baked potato topped with 1 teaspoon fat-free sour cream and 2 teaspoons trans free margarine, and 2 cups cooked broccoli. For dessert, have $^1/_2$ cup sorbet.

501 cal, 34 g pro, 73 g carb, 9 g fat, 3 g sat fat, 54 mg chol, 8 g fiber, 185 mg sodium, 119 mg calcium

Diet Exchanges: 0 milk, 1.5 vegetable, 0 fruit, 3.5 starch/bread, 3 meat, 1 fat

Take Your Pick: 200-Calorie Snacks

Skip the snack on days when you don't exercise or if you want to speed your weight loss. Be sure to factor the carbohydrates into your overall diet.

Fruit and Yogurt: Top $^1/_2$ cup cantaloupe cubes with 4 ounces ($^1/_2$ cup) fat-free lemon yogurt.

138 cal, 7 g pro, 28 g carb, 0.5 g fat, 0 g sat fat, 2 mg chol, 1 g fiber, 97 mg sodium, 226 mg calcium

Diet Exchanges: 0 milk, 0 vegetable, 0.5 fruit, 1.5 starch/bread, 0 meat, 0 fat

Cherries and Chocolate: Have $1^1/_2$ cups fresh Bing cherries with 1 bite-size dark (.25 ounce) chocolate candy.

128 cal, 2 g pro, 28 g carb, 2.5 g fat, 1 g sat fat, 1 mg chol, 3 g fiber, 0 mg sodium, 20 mg calcium

Diet Exchanges: 0 milk, 0 vegetable, 1.5 fruit, 0 starch/bread, 0 meat, 0 fat

Quick Pizza: Top half of a 100% whole wheat English muffin with 3 tablespoons low-sodium marinara sauce and 2 tablespoons shredded low-fat mozzarella cheese. Broil until cheese bubbles. Serve with 4 ounces orange juice or sparkling water over crushed ice.

174 cal, 8 g pro, 29 g carb, 3.5 g fat, 1.5 g sat fat, 9 mg chol, 3 g fiber, 282 mg sodium, 219 mg calcium

Diet Exchanges: 0 milk, 1.5 vegetable, 1 fruit, 1 starch/bread, 0.5 meat, 0 fat

Cookies and Milk: Eat 1 whole wheat fig bars with 1 cup 1% milk.

162 cal, 9 g pro, 25 g carb, 2.3 g fat, 1.6 g sat fat, 12 mg chol, 1 g fiber, 132 mg sodium, 290 mg calcium

Diet Exchanges: 1 milk, 0 vegetable, 0 fruit, 1 starch/bread, 0 meat, 0 fat

Veggies and Dip: Slice 1 red bell pepper into strips, and dip it and 10 baby carrots into $^1/_3$ cup store-bought hummus.

204 cal, 8 g pro, 27 g carb, 8.4 g fat, 1 g sat fat, 0 mg chol, 15 g fiber, 398 mg sodium, 72 mg calcium

Diet Exchanges: 0 milk, 2.5 vegetable, 0 fruit, 1 starch/bread, 0 meat, 1.5 fat

Cheese and Crackers: Have 1 piece low-fat string cheese, 3 low-sodium whole wheat crackers, and 1 medium apple.

185 cal, 9 g pro, 28 g carb, 5 g fat, 2 g sat fat, 0 mg chol, 5 g fiber, 31 mg sodium, 219 mg calcium

Diet Exchanges: 0.5 milk, 0 vegetable, 1 fruit, 0.5 starch/bread, 0 meat, 0.5 fat

Trail Mix: Mix $^1/_2$ cup Cheerios with 1 ounce almonds (approximately 22 nuts) and 1 teaspoon raisins.

233 cal, 8 g pro, 19 g carb, 16 g fat, 1.5 g sat fat, 0 mg chol, 5 g fiber, 106 mg sodium, 127 mg calcium

Diet Exchanges: 0 milk, 0 vegetable, 0 fruit, 1 starch/bread, 1.5 meat, 2.5 fat

Popsicles and Cookies: Enjoy 1 frozen 100% fruit juice bars and 1 small oatmeal cookie.

128 cal, 2 g pro, 25 g carb, 2 g fat, 0.5 g sat fat, 1 mg chol, 1 g fiber, 5 mg sodium, 17 mg calcium

Diet Exchanges: 0 milk, 0 vegetable, 0 fruit, 1.5 starch/bread, 0 meat, 0.5 fat

PB and Pineapple: Top 1 slice 100% whole wheat toast with 1 tablespoon peanut butter and $^1/_3$ cup pineapple chunks.

207 cal, 8 g pro, 25 g carb, 9 g fat, 2 g sat fat, 0 mg chol, 4 g fiber, 220 mg sodium, 49 mg calcium

Diet Exchanges: 0 milk, 0 vegetable, 1 fruit, 1 starch/bread, 1 meat, 1.5 fat

Strength-Train A: Core Control

Rollover Lift

TONES BACK, ABS, AND BUTT

Lie facedown, arms overhead. Lift your arms, head, and chest 2 to 4 inches off the floor. Hold for 1 count; lower, repeat once, then roll onto your back, lift your head and shoulder blades 3 to 4 inches, and reach toward your feet. Hold for 10 counts for 1 rep.

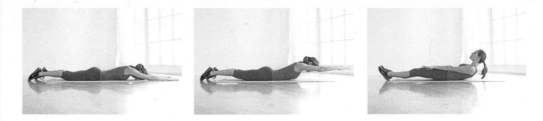

Make it harder: While facedown, lift your legs 3 inches off the floor as you lift your upper body.

Bridge with Fly

TONES CHEST, SHOULDERS, LEGS, BUTT, AND ABS

Holding a dumbbell in each hand, lie faceup with your upper back and head on a chair or bench, your knees over your ankles. Raise the dumbbells, keeping your arms straight, palms facing in. With your abs tight and hips lifted, lower your arms out to the sides until they are level with your shoulders. Raise your arms, squeezing your chest muscles, for 1 rep.

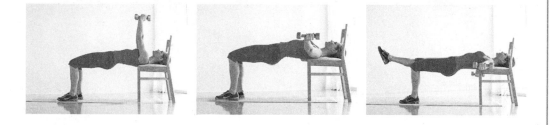

Make it harder: Extend your right leg so it's parallel to the floor. Switch legs halfway through reps.

Plank with Leg Raise

TONES CHEST, ARMS, ABS, AND BUTT

Place your hands shoulder-width apart on a chair or bench, with your arms straight, feet hip-width apart, and body aligned from head to heels. Keeping your abs tight, raise your right leg 6 to 12 inches off the floor, squeezing your glutes. Hold for 1 count, then lower. Alternate legs for 1 rep.

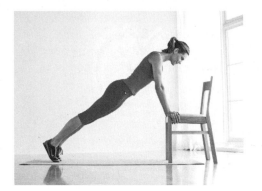 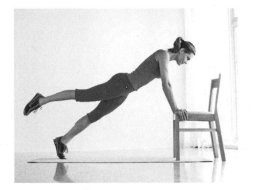

Make it harder: Bend your elbows and lower into a pushup. Holding the down position, raise and lower your right leg, and then push back up.

Core Reach

TONES ABS AND BACK

Lie faceup with your legs extended toward the ceiling, your arms overhead with palms up. Contract your abs as you raise your head and shoulder blades off the floor. Reach your hands toward your feet. Hold for 1 count, then lower.

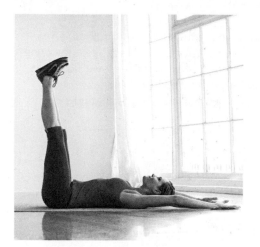 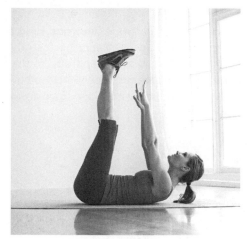

Make it harder: As you reach your hands toward your feet, lift your hips a couple of inches off the floor.

Strength-Train B: Butt Camp

Plié Extension

TONES BUTT, LEGS, INNER THIGHS, AND TRICEPS

Stand with your feet wide, toes out. Hold a dumbbell with both of your hands, arms overhead, palms up. With your back straight and abs tight, bend your knees, lowering until your thighs are almost parallel to the floor. Your knees should be over your ankles. At the same time, bend your elbows to lower the weight behind your head, keeping your upper arms close to your ears. Stand up while raising the weight for 1 rep.

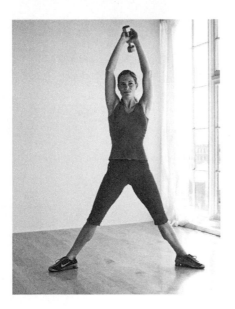 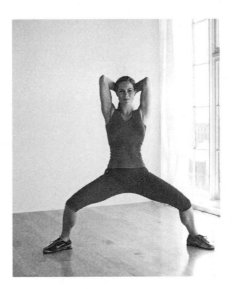

Make it harder: Do the move with a dumbbell in each hand.

Pelvic Lift

TONES HAMSTRINGS AND BUTT

Lie faceup with your left heel on a chair, knee slightly bent, and right leg extended toward the ceiling. With your arms at your sides, press your heel into the chair and squeeze your glutes to lift your hips as high as possible. Lower your hips about an inch from the floor for 1 rep. Switch legs halfway through the set.

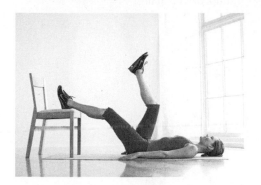 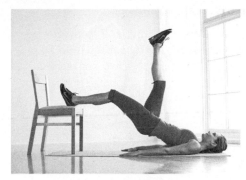

Make it harder: Squeeze a small ball or rolled-up towel between your thighs to engage your inner-thigh muscles.

Lunge with Curl

TONES LEGS, BUTT, AND BICEPS

Stand with your feet hip-width apart, holding dumbbells at your sides, palms forward. Step your right foot forward about 2 to 3 feet, lifting your left heel. Bend your knees and lower until your right thigh is almost parallel to the floor, with your right knee over your ankle. At the same time, curl the dumbbells toward your shoulders. Lower the weights as you press into your right foot and stand back up. Alternate legs for 1 rep.

Make it harder: Bring your back foot forward to meet your front foot, then step forward with the foot that was in back.

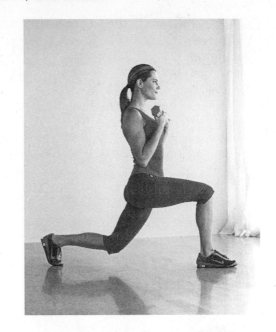

T-Chair

TONES LEGS, BUTT, AND SHOULDERS

Hold a dumbbell in each hand and stand with your back against a wall, with your feet 1 to 2 feet from the wall and about 6 inches apart. With your arms at your sides, palms in, bend your knees, squatting until your thighs are parallel to the floor, with your knees over your ankles. Holding the squat, raise your arms out to your sides to shoulder level, then lower, for 1 rep.

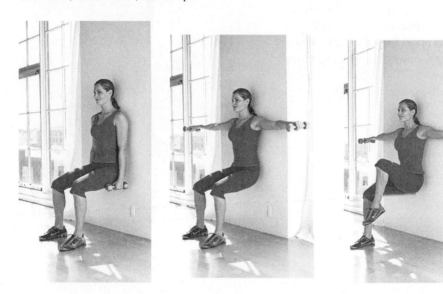

Make it harder: Lower into a squat, then lift your left foot several inches as you do arm raises. Switch feet halfway through reps.

CHAPTER 12

SMART CELEBRATING

12 real-world tactics for dealing with the number one overeating season

Many people have mixed feelings about this time of year—perhaps it's because the festive season is never just one upbeat note. It's never only happy, only loving, only blazing fires and cherub-cheeked children. The holidays, like life itself, are equally miserable and joyful, filled with both light and shadow. The problem is that we often forget the bad stuff. We forget that last year's family gathering was a semidisaster and believe that this year will be different. We get our hopes up. We enter the holidays with unrealistic expectations of how it's going to be and when it doesn't turn out that way, we often use food to comfort ourselves.

The holidays are a challenging time, and maybe you—like many of us—use food to help yourself cope. But after the food is gone, whatever causes you to overeat is still there. Food is only pleasurable, only delicious, only satisfying when you are hungry. In every other situation, something besides eating will comfort you and give you peace. Here are four holiday overeating triggers with strategies for surviving with your sanity—and waistline—intact.

TRIGGER: GOING HOME MAKES YOU ACT LIKE A CHILD

Every time Zoe walks in the door of her mother's house, she stops being an adult and feels about 3 feet tall. "I'm a grown woman, happily married, yet after spending 5 minutes with my older brothers and parents, I feel like the dumb little girl with big buckteeth who always gets left out," Zoe says. "Then I mindlessly eat anything I can get my hands on—which is, unfortunately, a lot."

No matter how old you are, your relationships with your parents and siblings may seem like they're set in stone. You're always the nerdy one or the little sister or the "problem child." One way we deal with this feeling is to try to tune out. Or we revert to childhood behaviors or indulge in adult comforts such as overeating.

Trigger Guards

Remind yourself that you're an adult. When going to your parents' house, bring along photos, letters, anything that reinforces your connection with your grown-up self. Zoe could bring a gift from a friend so she could have a concrete, physical object to look at when she feels she is regressing.

Spend time alone with your husband or a friend. Go for a walk or a drive. Sneak into a quiet room and shut the door, but do it with someone from your adult life. This will help keep you grounded in the present.

BYO fresh vegetables. Moms love to have our favorites waiting for us when we arrive home. In Zoe's case, that means piles of cookies, cakes, her mom's special vanilla fudge, and no vegetables—unless you count sweet potatoes with marshmallows. She could bring her own healthy foods with her. It isn't easy, but by having a plan and following through with it, you can stay securely in the present and avoid sliding into old patterns and old ways of eating.

TRIGGER: YOU FEEL VULNERABLE ABOUT YOUR SIZE

Joan dreads her family's Christmas dinner because she's gained nearly 20 pounds since she'd seen them all last year. "I know my Aunt Mary will say something about my weight," Joan explains, "and because she's mostly deaf, she'll do it at the top of her voice. I'll be absolutely mortified, and I'll eat everything that doesn't eat me first."

Joan's weight and her aunt's lack of a social filter are not the real issues. What is: Joan's self-worth is tied up in a number on a scale, a problem that many women share with her. When you or someone else defines you by your dress size, you start believing that if you're heavy, you must not be special, intelligent, or worth the space you take up. Joan is completely focused on her fears about what people will say and what her weight gain means (i.e., that she'll always be fat, that she is doomed, unlovable, unforgivable). She needs to change her focus.

Trigger Guards

Understand that you're not what you weigh. The size of your body and your self-worth are simply not the same things. To break that association, you need to disregard the negative self-talk that's going on in your head.

Learn to recognize hunger cues—an emptiness or rumbling in your stomach. As you become more aware of what your body is telling you, you'll be better able to eat only when you're hungry and stop when you've had enough. Eating then becomes a physical activity, not an emotional one.

Have a retort ready. On a very practical level, Joan has to decide how to respond to her aunt's barbs. She could say in a calm, even voice that she finds comments on her body size unhelpful. Or she could handle the situation with humor and say, "You think this is a weight gain? You should have seen what I looked like 2 months ago!"

Change the focus of the conversation. The least confrontational and often best approach to fielding a hurtful comment is simply shifting the subject without going into any explanation. If Aunt Mary makes a crack about Joan's size, she could deflect it by immediately asking about her aunt's latest vacation. People love talking about themselves to a good listener.

TRIGGER: YOU'RE SURROUNDED BY TEMPTING FOOD

Before Christmas, Oona's office resembles the "big rock candy mountain." Last year she feared it would sink her diet efforts like a torpedo. "I was really taking care of myself," she says. "I ate only when I was hungry and ate just what my body wanted. But when everyone else started eating treats, I felt incredibly deprived if I didn't join in." Oona also didn't want to seem rude by rejecting the food so lovingly prepared by her co-workers.

Trigger Guards

Sample only the special stuff. There's a big difference between eating home-made rugelach made by your office mate's Great-Grandmother Sadie and a box of store-bought Santa cookies with sprinkles. Eat what will give you the most satisfaction.

Listen to your body before, during, and after you eat. If a cookie looks good to you, ask yourself: "Do I want it because I think it will curb my hunger or because I want to treat myself?" If you really are hungry, then eat it. Enjoy the taste, the texture, and the whole experience of devouring it. But be sure to pay attention to how you feel 10 to 15 minutes afterward. If you're tired, spacey, or depressed, it wasn't really a treat, was it?

Oona realizes that the holidays are always going to be a dance between tuning in to her body, its hunger, and its fullness and being part of the festivities of food around her. But now, she says, "I'm able to be more choosy about what I eat and also feel like part of the gang."

TRIGGER: YOU'RE SUPPOSED TO BE JOYFUL . . . BUT YOU'RE NOT

Last year, Melissa's best friend was killed in a traffic accident right before Thanksgiving. Even though some time has passed, Melissa still doesn't feel much like celebrating. In fact, seasonal images of happy families make her cry—and eat, in an effort to bury her feelings, which seem so out of place in the face of all that "joy to the world."

It's not unusual to have what are called anniversary reactions around the time of a loss. Nor is it uncommon to feel blue during the holidays because of family dramas and societal pressures to be happy. In both cases, you experience a disconnect between what you think you should be feeling and what you actually feel. Despite your grief, there are a number of steps you can take to get through—and even find meaning in—the holidays.

Trigger Guards

Take time for tears. Losing someone you love is huge, and the feelings need to be honored and given space. Melissa needs to allow herself to feel the loss. She has agreed to set a timer for 10 minutes, three times a day—and just lie on her bed and weep. "It's a relief to be able to express my feelings, as big and sad as they are," she says. "Putting a time limit on them also lets me pay attention to the rest of my life."

Find activities you can enjoy. Melissa knows she doesn't want to do anything that feels "holidayish," but there are other ways to keep busy and make sure she isn't spending all her time mourning. A few suggestions: going cross-country skiing, seeing a movie, or heading to a day spa for pampering.

Socialize on a small scale. Melissa realizes that being with a big group makes her feel lonely (and when she feels lonely, she eats more). She has decided that it is best for her to be with one person at a time, so instead of making the party rounds, Melissa celebrates by having quiet dinners with close friends and family members. By paying attention to her own needs for contact, Melissa is able to feel her grief and honor her loss but not become so swamped by sadness that she turns to food for solace.

CHAPTER 13

THE DIET DERAILMENT SURVIVAL GUIDE

Top weight loss gurus reveal their safe, quick slim-down fixes

It happens to the best of us. You're trucking along on your weight loss plan just fine, and then—whammo—something pleasant (such as a vacation to Disney World or a visit home) or something stressful (such as a vacation to Disney World or a visit home) throws you completely off track.

The truth is, this does happen to everyone, even to diet docs. And the diet docs know that sometimes it takes a little something extra—think of it like a kick-start—to get your diet back on track again. But don't be tempted by quick-fix weight loss gimmicks. Juice fasts, cabbage soup plans, and herbal fat-burning pills are still big no-nos. Instead, consider the following less-extreme methods used by the nation's top weight loss gurus. Their back-on-track strategies and weight maintenance secrets are safe, effective, and sure to work for you, too.

DIET DERAILMENT: VACATIONS

"I just gained 4 pounds in Paris," says Kara Gallagher, PhD, assistant professor of exercise physiology at the University of Louisville. "I walked everywhere—almost 30,000 steps a day—so I thought I could eat everything, even creamy cheeses and desserts at night. (I suspect the reason French women are thin is not because they're eating right; it's because they smoke!) In the end, I was still consuming more than I could burn off."

Get-Back-on-Track Strategy

Salads—they're the perfect antidote to a week of no-holds-barred eating. "I also ban desserts, so if my sweet tooth is aching, I'll eat strawberries, raspberries, kiwifruit, or melon, which curb my cravings for rich, high-calorie desserts," says Dr. Gallagher. "Starch is out, but protein is in; lean meats, fish, and yogurt promote weight loss because they sit in your stomach longer, so you tend to stay full longer. Another way to feel full on fewer calories is to keep fat between 20 and 25 grams a day. That's the equivalent of a few slices of avocado, a 4-ounce piece of salmon, and a handful of walnuts or almonds."

Maintenance Plan

"I weigh and measure the food I eat, so I don't overpour the olive oil, salad dressing, or wine," Dr. Gallagher says. "When we go out to eat, my boyfriend and I split an entrée (unless we're in Paris—hey, sometimes prix fixe meals are too good to pass up!). I also exercise 6 days a week: I tend to do a 40-minute run and some sort of weight training at the gym four times a week, and a mind-body fitness class, such as yoga or Pilates, once or twice a week."

DIET DERAILMENT: DRINKING

"A few years ago, I would frequently have one or two glasses of wine at night with dinner, at about 120 calories per glass," says Caroline M. Apovian, MD, director of the Center for Nutrition and Weight Management at Boston Medical Center. "Not coincidentally, I weighed 10 pounds more than I do now."

Get-Back-on-Track Strategy

Stop drinking empty calories. "I never drink soda, but I make sure I kick fruit juice and alcohol, too," says Dr. Apovian.

"Liquid sugar is not satiating, and your brain doesn't register that you've consumed calories the way it would if you actually ate food; cutting it out is the quickest, easiest fix I know."

Maintenance Plan

Exercise every day for at least an hour. "If I don't do that I know I'll blow up," says Dr. Apovian. "Luckily, I love physical activity, and because on a typical day I either run for 6 miles or swim for an hour, I don't worry about food. That's my secret: Work out like you were born to do it."

DIET DERAILMENT: CARBOHYDRATES

"I crave the Cuban food I grew up on: rice, beans, and fried bananas," says Oz Garcia, PhD, nutritionist and author of *Look and Feel Fabulous Forever*. "I also love high-quality chocolate desserts."

Get-Back-on-Track Strategy

A low-carb, high-seafood diet. "Fish is high in protein and low in saturated fat, and it's rich in a nutrient called dimethylethanolamine (DMAE), which is good for your brain," Dr. Garcia says. "I cut out all starch such as potatoes, bagels, cereal, and pasta. I grill fish, lobster, and shrimp in olive oil, because I don't worry if there's a little fat in my diet—as long as it's not saturated fat from butter or red meat. I'll balance the fish with a fresh Greek salad or a salad made with roasted vegetables and firm stir-fried tofu."

Maintenance Plan

Lots of simple, fresh ingredients and fewer processed foods. "If I'm craving starch, I'll have basmati rice or a seven-bean soup instead of bread, because these foods are lower on the glycemic index, meaning they'll stick with me longer," Garcia says. "I also try to keep up the fish diet by having sashimi [sushi without rice] for dinner a couple of nights a week. I reach for healthy snacks such as nuts and dried fruit. The linchpin of this whole routine is walking to and from work—4 miles a day—then heading to the gym two or three times a week for upper-body training and some ab work on a stability ball."

DIET DERAILMENT: STRESS

"When I'm overwhelmed, I munch mindlessly on snack foods like Hershey's

Kisses and pistachios, especially at night," says Madelyn Fernstrom, PhD, director of the Weight Management Center at the University of Pittsburgh Medical Center. "Then my pants get a little snug, and the number on the scale is the reality check I dread seeing."

Get-Back-on-Track Strategy

Structured eating instead of stressed snacking. "I make sure I'm sitting down to three complete meals, at more or less the same time each day, and two small snacks," Dr. Fernstrom says. "Spreading out my food intake throughout the day means I'm never ravenous. Speedy weight loss comes when I eat more fruits and vegetables and minimize starchy carbohydrates—even fiber-rich varieties like whole grains. The reason: The body needs more water to digest the nutrients in starch, so eating less of it creates a fluid loss, which means I'll lose a pound or two almost immediately. That's enough to give me a mental boost. Because I'm a night eater, I try to give myself a bit of a treat every night so that I don't feel deprived. One of my favorite evening treats is a 100-calorie package of microwave popcorn or chips, which I eat one by one."

Maintenance Plan

"I monitor my weight by tuning in to the difference between 'head hunger' and 'biological hunger,'" Dr. Fernstrom says. "Chances are, if I ate recently, it's the former and has a psychological cause: Am I bored? Stressed? Tired?

"I work to solve that problem without food."

DIET DERAILMENT: GOING HOME FOR A VISIT

"I've always been pleasantly plump, but after graduate school my body inflated," says Carolyn Williams, RN, a weight loss coach in the department of endocrinology at the Mayo Clinic in Scottsdale, Arizona. "I remade my life and lost half my body weight, but maintaining my new weight of 165 pounds is a constant challenge. Flying home is especially tough because eating is what my family always does together. As soon as I step into our rural Pennsylvania kitchen, memories of comfort food ignite my cravings, and before I realize it, my hand will be in the cookie jar and my sister will be bringing out double-fudge something. Then we'll head over to the all-you-can-eat buffet, and boom—I've gained back 5 pounds."

Get-Back-on-Track Strategy

Extreme portion control. "With every meal, I make sure I'm eating just enough protein to fit into the palm of my hand," Williams says. "Protein promotes weight loss because it's more satiating than carbs, and your body burns more calories digesting it. I'll also drink lots of water—at least 75 ounces a day. It doesn't always make me feel less hungry, but it does make me feel healthier, which, in turn, makes me desire wholesome food. I aim to consume about 500 calories a day less than normal, and I'll try to burn an extra 500 calories a day, which means I can probably lose almost 5 pounds in 2 weeks."

Maintenance Plan

"I eat the foods that I love—like pizza—but I prepare them so that they're low in calories," Williams says. "After seeing a psychologist, I learned that I'd never be successful at maintaining my weight loss until I learned to work within what I like to eat. For example, Atkins didn't work for me. Now I know it's because I don't really like meat. I worry too much

about the cow that had to die to feed me. What I do like: bread and carbs. It took years, but I've finally come to terms with my need to eat pizza. But instead of ordering the heavily crusted kind that's brought to your door, I make it myself and load it with veggies. It's almost as easy and much healthier, but it also takes more forethought, which wards off mindless eating."

DIET DERAILMENT: BUSINESS TRAVEL

"Recently I went to California for a conference, and I started sneaking desserts and pasta with lots and lots of butter," says John Foreyt, PhD, director of the Behavioral Medicine Research Center at Baylor College of Medicine. "The extra calories and fat combined with no exercise had an immediate impact on my waistline."

Get-Back-on-Track Strategy

Meal replacements. "A 180-calorie Slim·Fast for breakfast, and, if I'm really in a hurry to lose, I'll have one for lunch, too," Dr. Foreyt says. "For dinner, I'll prepare a salad with oil and vinegar, a lean steak, and grilled vegetables.

"If I do that for a couple of weeks, I'll lose weight like gangbusters. Certainly, a lot of it is just water weight, but it will improve the way my clothes fit, and it's extremely motivating to see that number drop on the scale."

Maintenance Plan

"I like to have a Slim·Fast for breakfast because it's fast, preportioned calories," says Dr. Foreyt. "Then for lunch and dinner, I try to eat a normal, balanced meal, such as grilled chicken, a baked potato, and a vegetable and salad. I try not to have more than 2,200 total calories for the day.

"If I eat dessert one night, I make up for it by doing two meal replacements—using either Slim·Fast or a bowl of cereal—the next day."

CHAPTER 14

THE ROUND-THE-CLOCK FAT-BURNING PLAN

The new food, moves, and lifestyle tweaks that will keep your metabolism humming all day long

Metabolism is a mystery. You may know that mastering it is the key to losing weight, but what is it? And where is it? Turns out it's the engine that drives every cell, and that means it's everywhere. Your metabolism helps you walk, talk, fight off illness, even read this book. Its fuel: calories. Each one you consume goes into the metabolic tank that powers the machine that is you. Keep that tank filled and you're good to go, right?

If only it were that simple. As you age, your body becomes less effective at burning calories, mostly because of a gradual decrease in activity and resulting loss of muscle. Your metabolism can dip as much as 25 to 30 percent over your adult life, says Miriam Nelson, PhD, director of the John Hancock Center for Physical Activity and Nutrition at Tufts University. As a result, your body tends to store excess calories in the form of—you guessed it— body fat, and that extra weight only slows you down more.

You don't, however, have to resign yourself to a life of forgiving jersey fabrics and shape-disguising tunics. Strength-training increases the number of calories the body burns at rest, as much as 7 percent a day, by rebuilding muscle. You can increase it more by making small but targeted lifestyle changes.

"Anything that energizes you—a good night's sleep, fresh air, sunlight, a healthy diet, regular exercise—ultimately helps drive metabolism," explains Dr. Nelson.

With that in mind, we've designed a round-the-clock plan that will tune up your fat-burning engine, boosting its efficiency and maximizing calorie burn morning, noon, and night.

ALL-DAY METABOLISM MAKEOVER

By shifting your body into high gear, the following timely tips will help you burn 200 to 300 more calories a day. (And that doesn't even take into account your regular exercise routine.) Can't do it all? Don't worry—employing even a few of these steps will confer benefits. Now let's get going.

Morning

Here's how to get your day off to a fat-burning start.

Eat a 300- to 400-calorie breakfast. In the a.m., your energy stores are depleted by as much as 80 percent from the night before. Without food, your body shifts into starvation mode, which means it begins to conserve energy and burn fewer calories. (In other words: Your metabolic rate takes a nosedive.) That may be why, in one study, breakfast skippers were $4^1/_2$ times more likely to be obese than breakfast eaters. For more long-lasting energy, include whole grain complex carbohydrates such as oatmeal.

Throw in a cup of halved strawberries. Research suggests that getting enough vitamin C—75 milligrams a day—may be essential for optimal fat burning. The strawberries provide 90 milligrams.

Get a dose of sunlight. "Exposure to bright light decreases melatonin and increases serotonin, shifting your body from sleep to awake mode and, in turn, revving your metabolic furnace," says health and psychology researcher Robert K. Cooper, PhD, author of the metabolism book *Flip the Switch, Lose the Weight*.

Take your multivitamin. Antioxidant

nutrients help protect mitochondria, tiny structures found in every cell, from damage; they're the microscopic fat-burning furnaces that convert food into fuel.

Move at the office. "Moving throughout the day—even if it's just walking to a colleague's office rather than sending an e-mail—keeps your metabolism higher than doing a workout and then remaining sedentary," says James O. Hill, PhD, director of the Center for Human Nutrition at the University of Colorado Health Sciences Center.

Sip a cup of coffee or tea. Caffeine is a central nervous system stimulant that moderately boosts metabolism, helping you burn about 20 extra calories.

Have a midmorning snack. Good choices: a reduced-fat cheese stick or a cup of low-fat yogurt and a piece of fruit. Every time you eat, your body burns additional calories to digest the food. Take advantage of this automatic boost by eating something—even if it's very small—every 3 to 4 hours.

AFTERNOON

Keep your metabolism humming along through the middle of the day by following these tips.

Eat a protein-packed lunch. You'll burn more calories digesting your midday meal because protein is more difficult to break down than carbohydrates or fat. Here are three to try.

- Roast turkey breast with sliced veggies and hummus wrapped in a whole wheat tortilla; add a piece of fruit
- Salmon salad (similar to tuna salad but with canned salmon) topped with lettuce and tomato on a whole wheat bun; carrot sticks and grapes on the side
- Chicken-vegetable soup with a whole wheat roll

Snack on nuts. As your blood sugar and energy levels hit the postlunch slump, your metabolism also takes a dip. The protein and fiber in a handful of nuts (about 20) can help stave off hunger pangs and keep you energized until dinnertime. "Nuts also contain monounsaturated fats, which have been found in studies to stimulate fat burning," says Dr. Cooper.

Laugh it up. Laughing eases stress and boosts calorie burn up to 20 percent, reports a Vanderbilt University study of 90 men and women. Need a little inspiration? Check out www.theonion.com, an irreverent—and completely fake—news site.

(continued on page 140)

Your Morning Routine: Energizing Yoga

Accelerate the natural metabolic boost that occurs when you wake up by doing these poses. Yoga can also help control levels of the stress hormone cortisol, which begins to rise after waking and can contribute to muscle loss and a resulting dip in metabolism.

Downward-Facing Dog

Kneel with your hands directly beneath your shoulders, knees beneath hips, and toes tucked. Press your palms into the floor and lift your tailbone toward the ceiling, straightening your legs so your body forms an inverted V. Keep your shoulders away from your ears and relax your head between your arms. Hold for three to five breaths. Bend your knees and relax down to the floor.

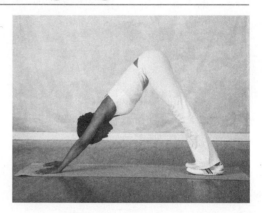

Cobra

Lie facedown with your legs extended, toes pointed. Place your hands on the floor beneath your shoulders, elbows close to torso. Press your feet, thighs, hips, and pelvis firmly into the floor and partially straighten your arms, lifting your chest as high as comfortably possible. Keep your shoulders down and back, lifting through your breastbone, opening your chest, and lengthening your spine. Hold for three to five breaths. Tuck your toes under and push back into Downward-Facing Dog. Repeat the moves three to five times.

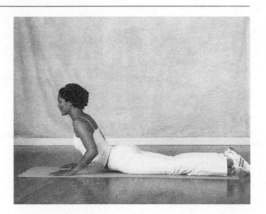

Take the stairs. Climbing stairs quickly elevates your heart rate for a metabolic jolt that burns 8 calories per minute—twice as much as brisk walking. Try to accumulate 5 to 10 minutes during the afternoon.

Brew some green tea. Studies show that the polyphenol compounds in 2 to 4 cups may help raise metabolism by as much as 35 percent and encourage fat burning.

Commute—with a CD. Relaxing music has been shown to reduce cortisol, a key metabolism-tempering hormone. Once tension has been tamed while on the highway, switch to more energizing music; upbeat tempos raise your heart and breathing rates and metabolism. And you'll be ready to tackle whatever awaits you when you arrive at home.

EVENING

Here's how to keep maxing your caloric burn as day turns into night.

Have a light (500- to 700-calorie) dinner. A balanced meal, such as fish, chicken, lean meat, or soy with steamed or sautéed veggies and a side of beans and rice, will refuel you without slowing you down. "Pause 15 minutes before taking second helpings; a relaxed eating style will ensure you don't get over-stuffed," suggests Dr. Cooper.

Pay bills, sort mail, surf the Web, or knit. You'll burn up to 54 more calories per hour than if you simply sit guarding the remote. (Bonus: Your hands will be too busy to reach into a bag of chips or cookies.)

Drink warm milk. Some studies suggest that amino acids in dairy products help promote fat burning. (Stick to low-fat or fat-free to keep calories in check.)

Lower the thermostat to sleep better. Skimp on shut-eye and you'll not only feel sluggish the next day—making activity less attractive—but you'll also be more at risk of gaining weight. A new report from the Nurses' Health Study, which followed more than 68,000 women for 16 years, found that women who slept just 5 hours a night were 32 percent more likely to gain 30-plus pounds during adulthood than those who got 7 hours of shut-eye, even though the light sleepers typically ate less.

Your Midday Workout: Interval Spring Walk

As little as 30 seconds of high-intensity exercise—such as sprints—can spike levels of human growth hormone by a whopping 530 percent, British researchers report. This boost, in turn, helps build lean muscle and burn fat.

With our routine, you won't be working quite that hard, but you'll increase the intensity enough to enjoy a metabolic bump that will last several hours. Related Canadian research reveals that eight exercisers doing just four 30-second sprints three times a week for 2 weeks doubled their endurance in exercise tests and ramped up their mitochondria activity by 38 percent, meaning their muscles and cells could use more oxygen and burn more calories.

The following workout is based on a 1-to-10 scale of intensity, with 1 equivalent to sitting on the sofa and 10 equivalent to sprinting.

TIME	EXERCISE
Minutes 1–2	Walk at 4 or 5, gradually ramping up to 7.
Minute 3	Blast off for 30 seconds at 9 or 10, then taper down to 5 for 30 seconds.
Minutes 4–5	Walk at 4 or 5, gradually ramping up to 7.
Minute 6	Blast off for 30 seconds at 9 or 10, then taper down to 5 for 30 seconds.
Minutes 7–8	Walk at 4 or 5, gradually ramping up to 7.
Minute 9	Blast off for 30 seconds at 9 or 10, then taper down to 5 for 30 seconds.
Minutes 10–11	Walk at 4 or 5, gradually ramping up to 7.
Minute 12	Blast off for 30 seconds at 9 or 10, then taper down to 5 for 30 seconds.
Minutes 13–15	Cool down at 4 or 5.

Stretch at Your Desk

Counter the metabolism-depressing effects of midday stress by boosting circulation and easing upper-body tension. And take deep breaths while you stretch to provide cells with the energy-producing oxygen they need to burn fat.

Chair Reach and Drop

Sit on the edge of a chair, your feet flat, back straight. Extend your arms overhead, palms facing each other, and gently arch back as far as comfortable. Hold for 1 to 2 seconds, then sit back up and lower your arms out to sides.

Clasp your hands behind your back and lean forward from your hips, bringing your chest toward your thighs, arms toward ceiling. Hold 10 to 15 seconds. Release and repeat.

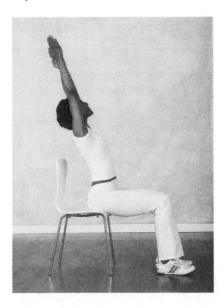 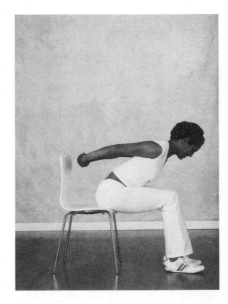

Your After-Work Exercise Plan: Strength-Building

"For every pound of muscle you build, you'll burn up to 50 extra calories a day," says Dr. Nelson. Why lift now? Body temperature inches upward as the day goes on, peaking around 5 p.m. (when it's about 1° to 2°F warmer than it is in the morning), priming your muscles for activity. Studies show that evening exercisers move faster, produce more power, and don't fade as fast—all while feeling less tired.

Try this multimuscle starter routine: Perform two sets of 8 to 10 reps 3 days a week, with a rest day after each.

Squat Press

Stand with your feet hip-width apart, abs tight. Hold 8- to 12-pound dumbbells by your shoulders, palms facing forward. Bend your knees and hips, lowering your body as if sitting into a chair—butt out, chest lifted, spine long. Keep your knees behind your toes and don't go lower than thighs parallel to floor. As you stand back up, press the weights overhead. Then lower them back to your shoulders and repeat.

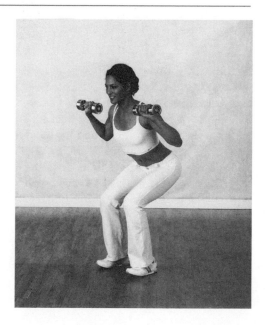

Lunge Curl

Stand with your left foot about 3 feet in front of your right, with left foot flat and right heel off the floor. Hold 8- to 12-pound dumbbells down at your sides, palms facing forward. Bend both knees, lowering your right knee straight down until your left thigh is parallel to the floor. Keep your left knee directly above your ankle. As you lower, curl the weights toward your shoulders. Then straighten your legs and lower the dumbbells back to start position and repeat.

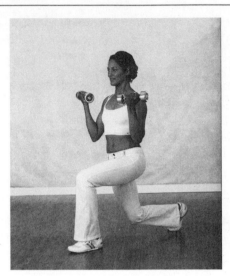

Plié Lat Raise

Stand with your feet wider than shoulder-width apart, toes pointing out. Hold 5- to 8-pound dumbbells down at your sides, palms facing in. Keeping your back straight, bend your knees and lower your hips until your thighs are nearly parallel to the floor. At the same time, raise the weights out to your sides until your arms are at shoulder height. Return to start and repeat.

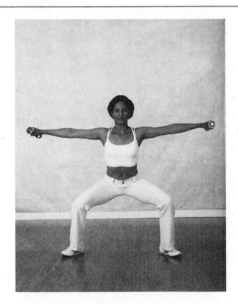

Calf Raise and Press

Stand with your feet close together and arms at sides, holding 5- to 8-pound dumbbells, palms facing in. Rise onto the balls of your feet, lifting your heels off the floor. At the same time, press your arms behind you, turning your wrists so your palms face the ceiling. Keep your arms straight. Lower and repeat.

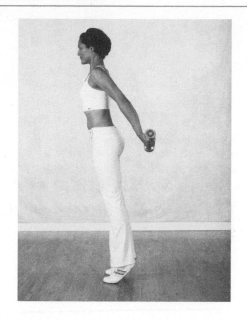

Curl and Press

Hold an 8- to 12-pound dumbbell in each hand and lie on the floor with your knees bent, feet flat. Position the dumbbells at either side of your chest, palms facing feet. Contract your abs and curl your head, shoulders, and upper back off the floor. Once in the up position, press the weights straight above your chest. Lower the weights, roll back to start, and repeat.

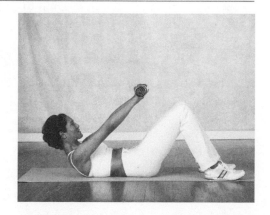

CHAPTER 15

PANTRY PSYCHOLOGY

One food scientist reveals why we eat as much
as we do—and offers 10 ways to stop ourselves

It's a typical Tuesday at the Food and Brand Lab at Cornell University, and director Brian Dr. Wansink, PhD, has invited some guests for lunch. The women think their free meal is a thank-you for testing the sound quality of iPods. But Dr. Wansink, one of the nation's few psychologists specializing in food marketing and eating behavior, has something else up his sleeve.

His grad students greet the guests, show them into the kitchen, and describe their lunch buffet: Royal Italian Bolognese, haricots verts, crusty bread with butter, and a beverage. Everyone eagerly starts serving themselves, not suspecting that they're being bamboozled by a scientific prank worthy of *Candid Camera*. Behind a one-way mirror, Dr. Wansink is watching them from his office as hidden cameras record all. Scales, hidden under dish towels on the counter, weigh how much food each person takes. "They're buying it," he says with a huge grin.

What they're buying is what they've been told: It's an elegant thank-you meal. But like anything that happens in Dr. Wansink's lab, nothing is what it seems. That Royal Italian Bolognese? It's really Beefaroni. The haricots verts? Canned green beans. This experiment is part of a larger test to see if people eat bigger portions when the food has evocative names. It's just one of hundreds he's conducted over the past 20 years in his lab, cafeterias, restaurants, and fast-food joints, trying to answer the most critical question for dieters: Why do we eat as much as we do?

Dr. Wansink chronicles decades of his work in his new book, *Mindless Eating.* And here, he shares 10 top eat-smarter tricks that really work.

CREATE STOP SIGNS

Dr. Wansink invited more than 100 women to view a video and rate it, but the real goal was to find out how many potato chips they'd eat while watching the TV. Everyone received a full canister of chips, but only one group got ordinary Pringles. The other groups got doctored packages: Either every 9th or every 13th chip was dyed red. Those with the regular Pringles ate 23, on average, while those with a dyed chip ate 10 or 15, respectively.

What's going on? Mindless munching. "The women got caught up in the video—not paying attention to how much they were eating—until something broke their rhythm," says Dr. Wansink. In this case, it was the red chip, but you can create your own natural break. "I portion out a snack on a plate or in a plastic bag and leave the rest in the kitchen," says Dr. Wansink. "I may get up for seconds, but I'll have to make a conscious effort to do so." (As some of his other studies show, you're far less likely to go back for more if you have to walk a couple of steps for it than if you have the package in front of you.)

If you absolutely must dig your hand into a bag, pick up single-serve packages, such as Nabisco 100 Calorie Packs or Orville Redenbacher's Mini Bags, which contain 110-calorie portions of popcorn.

IGNORE THE HEALTH HALO

Using a similar setup, Dr. Wansink asked another 100 or so women to his lab to watch a video and gave them same-size packages of low-fat granola to nosh on. The trick? Only half were labeled low-fat—and the women who got those ate 49 percent more (an extra 84 calories) than those whose bags bore no health claim.

What's going on? "Many people think low-fat means low-cal," he explains. "We assume that if a food is healthy in one way, it's good for us in all ways." That's how we get tricked by what Dr. Wansink calls health halos: the growing number of claims on food packaging trumpeting the lack of fat, the gobs of fiber, or the illness that the food prevents. Although all these assertions may be true, it's calories that count if you're trying to lose weight. After all, a trans-free doughnut still contains about 200 calories more than you can probably afford. So bypass such claims and head straight to the calorie info on the label to determine if a food really is diet-friendly.

FIXATE ON FULLNESS

In another sneaky study, 54 college students showed up to rate the quality of cafeteria food. Instead, each was served an 18-ounce bowl of Campbell's tomato soup. Some bowls were rigged to food-grade rubber tubing that snaked under the table and connected to a 6-quart soup vat that constantly refilled the bowl.

(Surprisingly, only one student caught on to the bottomless-bowl-of-soup trick.) After 20 minutes, students with the automatically refilling soup bowls ate an average of 15 ounces of soup, while the other students consumed about 9 ounces—a 135-calorie difference.

What's going on? Most people will eat what's put in front of them, stopping or slowing down only when a bowl is almost empty or when most of the food on the plate is gone. Hunger doesn't enter into it.

"I think the stomach has three settings," says Dr. Wansink. "They're 'I'm stuffed,' 'I'm full, but I could eat more,' and 'I'm starving.' Your goal is to recognize when you're full and not eat more." Don't rely on the amount of food left on your plate to signal when you're full. Instead, listen to your body's cues.

LEAVE THE MESS

Dr. Wansink is a real party animal. For one study, he invited 53 guests to a sports bar for a Super Bowl bash, during which he served free chicken wings and soft drinks. Waitresses were told to take away wing remnants from only half of the tables. The guests at the clean tables ate seven chicken wings, on average—two more than those whose tables held the visual proof of what they'd eaten.

What's going on? Unless you can see the damage, you're not going to remember how much you ate—and you'll eat more. A cluttered, messy table reminds you that you've eaten plenty. "At dinner parties, my wife and I often don't clear empty wine bottles from the table so we don't overindulge," he says.

HIDE YOUR TREATS

During Administrative Professionals Week one year, Dr. Wansink and another researcher gave out clear or white candy dishes filled with 30 Hershey's Kisses to the secretarial staff at the University of Illinois at Urbana-Champaign, where he was once simultaneously professor of business administration, nutritional science, advertising, and agricultural and consumer economics. A tag explained that the candy was a personal gift and requested that the employee keep it on her desk and not share it.

Dr. Wansink's ulterior motive: finding out whether the recipients would eat more from the bowls in which they could see the candy. Every night for 2 weeks, after the staff went home, he went from office to office, counting Kisses and refilling dishes. Those who got a clear dish ate eight pieces of candy every day, but those who got an opaque dish had about four—more than a 100-calorie difference.

What's going on? "We eat with our eyes," explains Dr. Wansink. "Having food in plain sight tempts people to eat every time they look at it." But surprisingly, that doesn't mean Wansink wants you to keep your kitchen and office junk-food free. "That only makes you feel deprived," he says. "When you're feeling deprived, your diet is doomed." Instead, keep small amounts of your favorite treats in the house, but hide them out of sight and out of easy reach—in an opaque container on a high shelf, at the back of the pantry, or in a distant room.

"I stash a couple of bottles of Coke in my refrigerator in the basement," says Wansink. "It's a hassle to run down there and get it when I want a bottle, so I don't do it that often." Conversely, keep healthy snacks where you can see and grab them. When you get a sugar jones, you can reach for that luscious pear on your desk or a banana from the glass bowl on the dining room table.

POUR SMARTER

Dr. Wansink and his crew went into bars in Philadelphia and asked the bartenders to pour a standard $1\frac{1}{2}$-ounce shot of whiskey or rum into either a tall, skinny 11-ounce highball glass or a short, fat 11-ounce tumbler. The pros were on target for the highball glasses but overpoured by 37 percent into the tumblers—even when asked to take their time. The point: "If bartenders can't pour the right amount, what hope do you have?" says Dr. Wansink.

What's going on? It's a trick of the eye; we tend to perceive objects that are tall as larger than short, squat ones. That means you're more likely to fill a low, wide juice glass to the brim but stop about halfway for the tall highball glass, even if they hold the same amount of liquid. So replace any short, wide glasses with tall, slim ones. Likewise, balloon-like red wineglasses can trick you into serving yourself more than the recommended 5 ounces a day.

"My wife wasn't happy about it, but we got rid of all the red wineglasses that we received for our wedding," says Dr. Wansink. And there are no juice glasses in his house, either.

KNOW WHERE YOU OVEREAT

When moviegoers in Chicago went to a 1 p.m. flick, Dr. Wansink and his colleagues gave them a treat—free medium or large buckets of popcorn—if they were willing to answer "concession-related" questions after the film. But this treat was a trick—the popcorn was stale. Most people reported that it tasted bad. Despite that and the fact that they'd eaten lunch before the movie, the average patron consumed more than 250 calories' worth of stale popcorn—more if they received a large container.

What's going on? You may be more influenced by where you are (at the movies), what you're doing (sitting in the dark, watching an engrossing flick), and what the people you're with are doing (also chomping away) than by the taste and quality of the food in front of you or your own hunger. That's why you'll have popcorn at the movies, hot dogs at the ballpark, and ice cream on a hot summer night, no matter how they taste or how full you are. If you find that you're tempted, have a bottle of water or pop a piece of sugar-free gum as a substitute.

SERVE SMALL

Forty graduate students showed up for a Super Bowl party that Dr. Wansink threw on the pretense that he was studying the new commercials. The real deal: By using a scale hidden under a tablecloth, his crew weighed how much Chex Mix guests took from either half-gallon- or gallon-size bowls. He discovered that the students who served themselves from the gallon bowl took 53 percent more than those who served themselves from the smaller bowl.

What's going on? "We use background objects as a benchmark for estimating size," says Dr. Wansink. "If all the serving bowls are big, what ends up on our plate is a big portion." That's why you should stick to serving bowls that hold just 4 to 6 cups of food. And scale down everything else: Portion out the food with a tablespoon rather than a much-larger serving spoon, and, as he did, switch to salad plates in place of Frisbee-size dinnerware.

RATE THE TASTE

Guests at the Spice Box in Illinois—a testing ground for wannabe chefs—received a free glass of wine with their meals, courtesy of Dr. Wansink. Tables on the right side of the room were offered their drink from "a new winery in California"; the left side got theirs from "a new winery in North Dakota." Except for this wording, both labels were identical. In reality, all of the wine was the ultracheap Charles Shaw brand—often referred to as Two Buck Chuck—from Trader Joe's. All guests could order whatever they wanted off the same menu. Those who received the California wine ate, on average, 11 percent more of their food than those who got the North Dakota vintage.

What's going on? "Once patrons saw the wine was from California, they said to themselves, 'This meal is going to be good,'" says Dr. Wansink. "And once they concluded that, their experience lined up to confirm their expectations."

A great rating, fancy tableware, a prestigious label—or a free glass of wine or appetizer—doesn't guarantee quality. Imagine you're a restaurant reviewer, and critically examine the flavor of whatever you eat. If you don't care for the dish, don't finish it. And if your whole meal has been only so-so, don't take a chance on dessert. Ask yourself, "Is this really worth the calories?" If it isn't, stop eating.

KEEP SNACKS SIMPLE

PTA parents attending a special meeting to view a video each received a bag of M&M'S. Though the bags were the same size, the M&M'S inside were different: Some of the packages contained 7 colors, while others had 10. Those with the most colorful candies ate a whopping 43 more candies than those whose bags held fewer hues.

What's going on? "When there's a variety of foods—even if the difference is as subtle as the color of M&M'S—people want to try them all," Dr. Wansink says.

"So they end up eating more—a lot more, in fact."

Use variety to your advantage. Keep seven or eight different kinds of fruits and veggies in the house rather than three or four. Look for prepackaged produce that offers variety. But when it comes to high-cal, high-fat treats, keep choices to a minimum. If you must have M&M'S, stock up on holiday versions, which usually contain only two or three colors.

And what about the women who ate the fake Bolognese for lunch? Those who thought the Beefaroni was a gourmet feast ate considerably more than those who were told that lunch came from a can. One woman even said, "It was the best lunch I had all week."

MEDICAL BREAKTHROUGHS

Here's the newest research on the weight loss front.

GET SLIM TO OUTWIT DIABETES PAIN

About 41 million US adults have prediabetes: higher-than-healthy blood sugar levels that don't quite qualify as diabetes. And although people with prediabetes might not realize it can happen, some will suffer tissue damage that's more common in the full-blown disease: death of small nerves in the hands and feet, causing chronic pain. But University of Utah research found that losing just a little weight may actually regenerate those nerves.

The good news: After 1 year, pain disappeared in 22 out of 32 people with prediabetes who lost 7 percent of their body weight through healthy eating and exercise. Biopsies taken at the beginning and the end of the study showed that nerve fibers increased by 33 percent at one spot on the calf and 29 percent at another spot on the thigh in all the participants.

Here's why it works: Lowering body fat helps lower blood sugar levels. Elevated levels have been found in other research to damage tiny nerve endings.

SHRINK YOUR WAIST

Diet and exercise are a dynamic duo—the combination will shrink abdominal fat cells, too many of which raise your risk of diabetes and heart disease. Wake Forest University researchers asked 45 obese women to start a diet; two-thirds of them also walked three times a week at either a slow pace for 55 minutes or a slightly faster one for 30 minutes. After 20 weeks, everyone had lost about 25 pounds. But the walkers also reduced the size of their abdominal fat cells by 19 percent. The diet-only women had no such change. This isn't power walking either: The faster group kept a very manageable 3 to 4 mph pace; the slower ones walked half that fast.

TAKE THE FAST LANE TO WEIGHT LOSS

Start ringing up your own groceries: According to an IHL Consulting Group survey of 533 consumers, women who use the self-checkout lane are about half as likely to make impulse buys that could add pounds. Your savings: 7,200 calories a year—2 pounds of weight gain.

TRICK YOURSELF THIN

Midafternoon, you have chips from the vending machine. Half an hour later, you're munching pretzels. If instead you ate foods that you associate with meals— a hard-cooked egg or a turkey-and-cheese roll-up—you'd feel full longer, say scientists from the University at Buffalo, the State University of New York.

Their study found that undergrads who labeled midafternoon treats as "snacks" ate 87 percent more at dinner than those who ate identical 2:30 p.m. foods but classified them as "meals." If you choose items that you think of as meals—real food, rather than treats— they'll more likely satisfy your appetite, says lead researcher Elizabeth D. Capaldi, PhD.

Kathy McManus, RD, director of the nutrition department at Brigham and Women's Hospital in Boston, developed these healthy meal-for-snack swaps for *Prevention* at two calorie levels. Choose a 150-calorie minimeal if you normally eat three substantial meals and two snacks every day; the 250-calorie options are for those who usually spread their daily calories over five or six small meals.

150 Calories

Instead of this snack: 6 ounces fruited fat-free yogurt

Eat this "meal": $^1/_2$ small whole wheat pita, 2 thin slices turkey breast, sliced tomato, and mustard

Instead of this snack: 1 ounce pretzels and $^1/_2$ cup grapes

Eat this "meal": $^1/_2$ whole wheat English muffin, 1 ounce reduced-fat mozzarella cheese, and green bell pepper and tomato slices

250 Calories

Instead of this snack: energy or breakfast bar

Eat this "meal": 1 slice whole wheat toast, 1 scrambled egg, and 2 slices turkey bacon

Instead of this snack: trail mix with chocolate chips, cashews, and dried fruit

Eat this "meal": whole wheat tortilla, slice of avocado, 2 slices chicken breast, tomato, lettuce, and 1 tablespoon salsa

DROP 3 POUNDS WITHOUT TRYING

Put that cola down! And head for the sink instead. According to a study of 240 overweight women conducted by the Children's Hospital and Research Center in Oakland, California, dieters who swap sugary beverages for water lose an extra 3 pounds a year, on average, compared with those who continue to chug the sweet stuff. Sure, cutting out soda saves calories, but it's possible that water helps rev your metabolism, because well-hydrated cells may process carbs and fat more efficiently.

TURN OFF THE TUBE

We've all heard the news that too much TV time can make you, well, fat. But according to a study in the journal *Obesity*, too many hours in front of the TV can also make it harder to maintain weight loss.

Researchers analyzed data from 1,422 people enrolled in the National Weight Control Registry who had maintained a loss of at least 30 pounds for a year. They found that people who increased their TV time gained an average of 9 pounds, while those who cut back gained only 2. To keep lost pounds from creeping back, limit tube time to 10 hours weekly.

SCALE UP

Guesstimates work fine when you're making a stew but not when it comes to your weight. In a study in the *New England Journal of Medicine*, 209 women who'd lost an average of 20 percent of their body weight were assigned to either face-to-face meetings or an Internet program with the goal of regaining no more than 5 pounds. Researchers asked the women to weigh themselves weekly, but those who hopped on the scale every day were 82 percent less likely to bulk back up.

"Weighing daily keeps people vigilant," says study author Rena Wing, PhD. To keep off lost pounds, weigh in every morning. Up a pound or two? Hit the gym a couple more times and skip dessert that week. If you go above 3 pounds, return to your original diet.

HAVE A CUPPA

One more reason to drink tea: Compounds in black, green, and mulberry teas may prevent our bodies from absorbing calories from carbohydrates, according to research in the *American Journal of Clinical Nutrition*.

In the study, 20 people ate a meal of white rice with a beverage—either a combination of the three tea extracts or a placebo liquid. Researchers then measured the subjects' breath hydrogen levels, which indicate whether carbohydrates are being digested; the levels were higher when the people drank tea.

In fact, "25 percent of the calories in the meal were not absorbed by the tea drinkers," says study author Michael Levitt, MD. "More studies are needed, but you could lose 16 to 18 pounds a year if you drink these teas after every meal."

SAY YEAH FOR CLA

Don't sweat those pieces of candy you enjoyed from your co-worker's candy dish. A study hints that a pill can keep those treats from threatening your waistline. University of Wisconsin researchers gave 40 overweight subjects either 4 grams a day of a supplement called conjugated linoleic acid (CLA) or a placebo. No one was dieting, but after 6 months, those who'd taken CLA had lost 1.3 pounds, while those in the placebo group gained 2.4. The most substantial differences were seen during the holiday months: The placebo poppers put on more than a pound each, but members of the CLA group took off about a third of a pound from November through December.

"CLA increases the burning of fat, particularly during sleep," says study coauthor Dale Schoeller, PhD. "The effect is very small but adds up over months—and because people tend not to notice gradual weight gain during the winter, every little bit can help."

CLA, a fatty acid, is naturally found in beef and dairy fat. You can get Tonalin, the capsule used in the study, at www.drugstore.com; volunteers took four 1,000-milligram pills each day with breakfast.

Success Story

She Refused to Deprive Herself

Debra Janney, 36, was 29 when her husband left. It was such a shock that she became depressed and stopped eating. She went from 110 pounds to 90. She was so preoccupied with the divorce and caring for her 2-year-old son, Truitt, that she didn't pay attention to what was happening to her.

After the divorce was finalized and Debra settled into life as a single mom, her depression started to lift and her appetite returned. Running after a toddler, working as an accountant, and taking care of a home kept her busy, so eating right was her last concern. She ate a lot of takeout and fast-food hamburgers and fries, doughnuts, and McDonald's Big Breakfast with scrambled eggs, sausage, hash browns, and a biscuit, and she regained the weight she had lost. But it didn't stop there. Within 2 years, she had packed on an extra 25 pounds.

Soon Debra's size-four pants made way for sixes. And then eights. As a single parent, it killed her to spend money on new clothes just because she had gained weight. When even her size eights became uncomfortable and she had to unbutton them while sitting at her desk at work, she decided it was time to act.

The Family Diet

When Debra was a kid, the women in her family were always dieting. But at family gatherings, they'd pile their plates high. The joke was: "I'll start my diet again on Monday." Monday would come and they'd try the latest fad diet, deprive themselves of their favorite foods, and eventually give up.

Debra didn't want to get stuck in her family's diet cycle, but she didn't want to give up her favorite foods either. "Let's face it: Sometimes a yummy dessert is worth the extra calories," she thought. But she was willing to start exercising.

(continued)

Success Story (cont.)

Her parents' treadmill was collecting dust, so she borrowed it and began walking a mile a day. She quickly became bored watching TV while she walked, but she stuck with it because she knew it was the only way she could eat what she wanted and still lose weight.

After a month, Debra invested in a CD player and discovered that walking was much more fun with music. Soon she was picking up the pace, adding mileage, and feeling more energetic. She eventually added an incline and some running. Within 3 months she had lost 10 pounds.

Sticker Shock

The treadmill inadvertently made Debra eat smarter, too, because she paid attention to its calorie counter. As she became more conscious of what she was putting in her mouth, she started to read food labels. One day she looked up her favorite McDonald's breakfast on the company Web site. It was 720 calories! She'd have to walk more than 7 miles to burn off just that one meal. It wasn't worth it. She didn't want to give up all her favorite treats, but she had to make wiser food choices if she wanted to lose more weight.

Debra was never a fan of fruits and vegetables, but everything she read recommended them because they're nutritious, high in fiber, and low in calories. So she gave them a shot. Apples weren't so bad. Then she tried plums and peaches. To her surprise, she liked them, too.

As the weight continued to melt away, Debra made another switch that paid off: bringing low-calorie frozen entrées and fruit to work instead of ordering greasy takeout. For quick dinners, she swapped regular burgers for lower-fat turkey burgers.

Weekend Rewards

To control her cravings, Debra made a deal with herself: If she ate sensibly during the week, she could indulge on the weekends. So when she'd see mouthwatering french fries on a commercial or watch her son devour a candy bar, She'd remind herself that she could have whatever she wanted, but she had to wait for the weekend. To make up for the extra calories, she was very active on Saturdays and Sundays. She'd hop off the treadmill and take longer walks or runs outside each day. She usually spent 3 hours cutting, edging, and blowing leaves off the lawn. Add in housecleaning—sweeping, mopping, vacuuming, and doing laundry—and she burned enough calories to have pizza with Truitt (she still added a side of veggies) and hot-out-of-the-oven chocolate chip cookies for dessert without feeling guilty.

Delaying her cravings helped Debra be more discriminating in what she ate. Sure, she wanted cookies, cakes, and chips during the week, but when the weekend rolled around, she'd find that she had narrowed the list to the indulgences that were really worth the calories. So instead of wolfing down a dozen store-bought cookies without actually tasting them, she'd savor every bite of the three or four homemade ones that she'd "earned."

It took 2 years, but Debra lost 25 pounds. And nothing felt as good as the moment she finally waltzed into the Gap to buy jeans in a smaller size. She pulled on the fours, but they were too big. The salesgirl gave her a size two, but they were baggy as well. The size ones fit just right—and 3 years later, they still do.

PART IV

MOVE IT!

CHAPTER 16

SIX WAYS TO DOUBLE YOUR RESULTS

Firm up faster with these ingenious ideas

No one has to be a slave to the gym to get a slimmer, sexier body. Not now. Not ever. Research proves it: You don't have to work out longer—just smarter. Make these easy tweaks to your routine and spend the time saved enjoying your svelte new shape.

POWER UP YOUR WALKS

Old thinking: Stretch first.
New approach: Get moving.

A review of 23 studies found that stretching before an activity damages muscle tissue, which reduces muscle strength and hinders performance. Start each workout by moving your limbs through a full range of motion, says certified personal trainer and walking coach Judy Heller of Portland, Oregon. "You want to get the fluid in your joints flowing, so your ankles, hips, knees, and shoulders are well lubricated and move with ease," she says.

Improve results: Do each of the following moves 6 to 10 times before you start walking. And stretch only after your workout. Studies show this can help keep you limber and prevent chronic injuries such as tendinitis.

Heel raise. Lift heels off ground, rising on toes, then rock back slightly onto heels so toes come off ground.

Four-way leg lifts. Shift weight to left leg and gently swing right leg out to side as far as it will go and then back across your body. Repeat with left leg. With weight on left leg again, raise right knee toward chest, then swing and extend it to back. Repeat with opposite leg.

Hula-hoop swivel. Rotate hips like you're hula-hooping. Reverse direction.

Shoulder swing. Keeping shoulders relaxed, bend elbows and gently swing arms forward and back, stretching through chest and fronts of shoulders.

BURN MORE FAT

Old thinking: Walk long and steady.
New approach: Do speed bursts.

Short pops of energy help your body burn fat both while you work out and long afterward—and in less workout time. In a recent study, exercisers who performed just 2 to 3 minutes of high-intensity, 30-second sprints on exercise bikes (with 4 minutes of easy pedaling in between) 3 times a week boosted their ability to use oxygen—a key factor in fat burning—by about 30 percent, says study author Martin Gibala, PhD, an associate professor of kinesiology at McMaster University in Ontario. What's more, your metabolism stays revved longer after a vigorous workout than after an easy one: Researchers from Canada's Laval University found that although participants who did short bursts burned only half as many calories during their workouts as peers who exercised longer, they had burned 9 times as much fat after 15 weeks.

Improve results: If you normally walk for 45 minutes, cut it down to 30. After a short warmup, speedwalk at your fastest pace for 1 minute. Recover for 1 minute, walking at a moderate pace. Repeat about 15 times. Cool down.

ERASE ARM, HIP, AND THIGH FLAB

Old thinking: Lift for 12 to 15 reps.
New approach: Pump out only 3 to 5.

Performing just a few reps with heavy weights activates hard-to-tone "fast-twitch" muscle fibers that atrophy (hence the jiggly flesh) as you age. Problem is, many women use 3- to 5-pound dumbbells when they really should be using 10-pound or even heavier weights, says researcher William Kraemer, PhD, a physiology professor at the University of Connecticut. If you amp up your weight-training, you can fire up those fibers and regain your strength and shape.

Improve results: Once a week (but no more—your muscles need to recover), trade in your 3- and 5-pound dumbbells for 10-, 15-, even 20-pounders or heavier. Think it's too hard? Remember, you routinely pick up 10-pound grocery bags and maybe even 50-pound kids. Shoot for three sets, 3 to 5 reps per set. If you can't maintain good form, the weight is too heavy; pick a slightly lighter one.

TIGHTEN YOUR ABS

Old thinking: Hit the mat.
New approach: Stand up.

Your abs are made of endurance-based muscle fibers, which is a fancy way of saying that it takes dozens of crunches to fatigue (and tone) them. However, many women who do crunches on the floor find that their necks start to ache before their abs begin to burn, so they stop—and never get the firm midsections they want. The secret to firmer, flatter abs: Add rotation—twisting your abs and obliques (side muscles)—to other strength moves such as squats or lunges. These muscles are designed to hold you upright and stabilize your torso, and anytime you twist or turn, they jump into action, says Andrew Fry, PhD, a professor of exercise and sport sciences at the University of Memphis. Activate them throughout your workout and they'll be quicker to fatigue once you hit the floor.

Improve results: When you do lunges, add a twist, rotating from your middle toward the knee that's out in front. Also, when you stand up from a squat, raise one knee toward the opposite shoulder as high as you can and rotate your torso toward that knee. Then, come crunch time, you can cut your repetitions in half.

DO ANYTHING BETTER

Old thinking: Dive right in.
New approach: Think first.

Scientists from the Cleveland Clinic found that when men and women simply imagined exercising their little fingers and biceps for 15 minutes a day, 5 times a week for 12 weeks, their strength increased by up to 35 percent—without actually moving a muscle. This is a testament to the power of the mind-muscle connection, says Sean McCann, PhD, sports psychologist with the US Olympic Training Center in Colorado Springs. "When you visualize an action, your brain develops a model of it that allows you to recruit the muscles you need and perform more effectively and efficiently when you actually do it," he says.

Improve results: Take a few seconds to picture yourself performing a perfect set of squats, executing a smashing tennis serve, or briskly walking down your favorite path. Then get out there and do it.

AVOID DROP-OUT-ITIS

Old thinking: Take time off.
New approach: Skip the rest days.

Exercise—even a light workout—actually reduces next-day soreness and speeds your body's recovery. The reason? It increases bloodflow, which delivers healing nutrients to your muscles and flushes out metabolic waste. Plus, "when you move your body every day, whether it's taking a walk, lifting weights, or simply stretching, exercise becomes part of your daily landscape, which means you're working out more consistently," says Steve Glass, PhD, a professor of exercise physiology at Grand Valley State University. "And that almost guarantees faster results." (Read: You'll burn more calories.)

Improve results: Do some activity every single day, even if it's only for 10 or 15 minutes. This doesn't have to mean more exercise. Simply borrow time from your other workouts and spread it out over the week.

Quick Tip

Count each completed repetition as one point, and after each exercise, tally your points. Aim to increase your total each workout, but don't sacrifice good form to do more reps.

CHAPTER 17

FIVE MOVES THAT FIRM

Burn calories, sculpt muscle, shed fat—and
you don't even have to leave your living room

Clothes feeling a little snug? We have the perfect fix: a workout that produces major results—namely, sexy shoulders, a flatter tummy, and a firmer butt and thighs—in 6 short weeks. Plus, "All of these exercises involve multijoint movements, so you're firming up individual muscles while training them to work together," says Benjamin Hendrickson, an American Council on Exercise–certified personal trainer at the Sports Center at Chelsea Piers in New York City, who designed this innovative strength-training circuit. That means better balance and more coordination, whether you're juggling clubs and balls on a golf course or a plate of stuffed mushrooms in one hand and a cocktail in the other at a party. Because you're moving your body weight instead of sitting stationary at a machine, you're also getting a metabolic boost. Best of all, you can do these moves in your living room. So get ready to slip into your favorite outfits once again with confidence!

STEPUP

Works glutes, quads, hamstrings, calves, and core

STAND in front of a staircase or step with your feet together, arms at sides. Place your left foot solidly on the step, keeping your head up and abs tight. Lift your body onto the step, raising your right knee until your thigh is parallel to the floor. Hold for a second. Lower your right foot to the floor behind the step, then lower your left. Repeat, stepping up with your right foot and raising your left knee. Continue alternating legs.

Why it works: In addition to mimicking real-life demands, such as climbing stairs, the stepup forces you to engage your core; raising the knee challenges your balance.

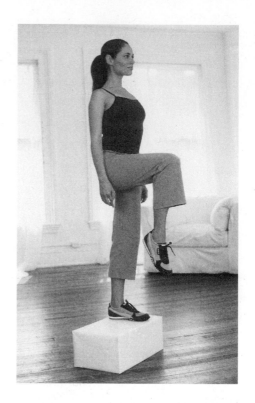

Workout Basics

The equipment: You'll need a kitchen timer or a clock with a second hand that you can easily see, along with either a staircase or an 8- to 12-inch step (beginners use a one-level step; advanced exercisers, a two-level version).

The routine: Warm up for 5 minutes by marching or jogging in place. Then do the five exercises, devoting 1 minute to each. Rest for 1 minute and repeat the circuit.

Beginners: Do three complete circuits.

Advanced: Do five complete circuits.

The plan: Do this workout three times a week on nonconsecutive days. Once a week, skip the timer and do 10 reps of each exercise, concentrating on form.

ELBOW-TO-KNEE SITUP

Works abs

Lɪᴇ on the floor with your knees bent, feet flat on the floor. Place your hands behind your head and lift your head and feet a few inches off the floor, pointing your elbows toward your knees. Contract your abdominals and rock up so your elbows meet your knees and you're resting on your "sitz" bones, literally the bones you sit on. Hold for a second, then lower. Keep your head and feet off the floor during the entire minute. If this is too challenging, keep your midback on the floor and lift your hips and shoulder blades to bring your knees and elbows together.

Why it works: Bringing your elbows to your knees forces you to coordinate your upper and lower body, increasing abdominal strength and body awareness.

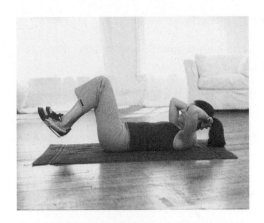

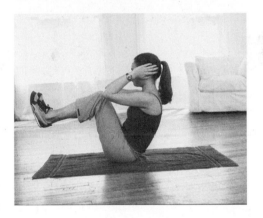

MOUNTAIN CLIMBER

Works glutes, quads, hamstrings, calves, core, and chest

ASSUME a pushup position, with your hands flat on the floor beneath your shoulders and your feet hip-width apart, balancing on your toes. Bend your right knee and plant the ball of your right foot beneath your torso. Spring off your toes and raise your hips into the air, switching legs, so your right leg is extended and your left leg is bent. Repeat, alternating legs.

Why it works: This oldie-but-goodie keeps your heart rate high, cranking up your calorie burn to melt fat.

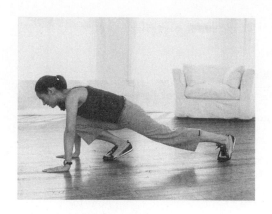

ROTATING SIDE LUNGE

Works glutes, quads, hamstrings, outer thighs, and obliques

STAND with your feet hip-width apart, your arms extended at chest level, and your hands clasped. Take a giant step to the left, rotating your upper body toward the left. Bend your left knee and lower your hips, keeping your left knee over your foot. Press into your left foot to return to the starting position and repeat. Do a full minute, then switch sides.

Why it works: This move forces you to balance and coordinate your upper and lower body while moving side to side. "It's a great exercise for strengthening muscles that often go underused in daily life," says Hendrickson.

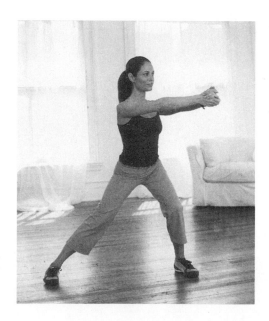

PUSHUP

Works chest, shoulders, triceps, and core

PLACE your hands on the floor beneath your shoulders and balance on your toes, with your feet hip-width apart. Bend your elbows out to the sides and lower your body almost to the floor. Keep your abs tight and your body in a straight line from head to ankles. Rest your knees on the floor, keeping your toes tucked, and push back up. At the top of the movement, straighten your legs and repeat.

Why it works: This hybrid of the standard pushup and the less-demanding knees-down version allows you to build upper-body strength quickly, for a flattering figure.

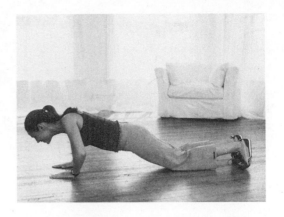

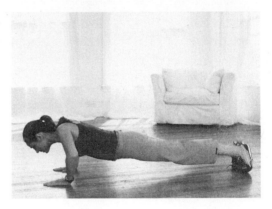

CHAPTER 18

6 WEEKS TO A TONED BODY

Say good-bye to belly fat with
high-energy walks, power Pilates,
and the best flat-abs foods

You exercise and eat right, but your waistline refuses to budge. Sound familiar? Sadly, after age 40 you need to work harder to whittle your middle. But with our science-backed three-part plan, you can get a flatter belly in 3 to 6 weeks (the bigger your bulge, the faster you lose).

A recent Skidmore College study shows that a program of challenging strength exercises, vigorous cardio, and a slight shift in food choices (not a diet!) cut twice as much abdominal fat as the typical low-fat and cardio plan, while slashing more than an hour a week off your workout. Our version combines ab-targeting Pilates moves, high-powered walks, and fat-busting foods to slim your midsection—and reduce your risk of diabetes, as well as heart disease and other life-threatening health issues.

You'll notice less allover jiggle in 3 weeks as you build muscle and shed fat. In 6 weeks, you'll trim inches off your waist, thanks to a loss of 10 to 12 pounds.

Keep going for a firmer stomach in about 6 months. Happier, healthier, stronger, slimmer: So this is life after 40!

POWER WALK

Improve your body's calorie-burning ability and shrink fat cells. Start with 20 minutes, but if you feel ready for more, go for it! The key is to walk with focus, pumping your arms and working every muscle, to maximize your calorie burn. Here's how.

Use your full stride. Land squarely on your heel, then roll through the foot to push off strong with the toes.

Make it brisk. Be sure to keep your breathing regular and controlled, but maintain a pace that makes it a little difficult to carry on a conversation.

Your Workout at a Glance

WEEK	1	2	3	4	5	6+
Power Walk (see above)	3 days: 20 min	3 days: 25 min	3 days: 30 min	3 days: 30 min	3 days: 30+ min	3 days: 30+ min
Triple-Decker Walk (see page 174)	1 day: 18 min	1 day: 24 min	1 day: 30 min	2 days: 18 min	2 days: 24 min	2 days: 30+ min
Pilates Power Moves (see page 174)	3 days: earlier versions or main moves	5 days: earlier versions or main moves	3 days: main moves	5 days: main moves	3 days: harder versions	5 days: harder versions

The Experts: Los Angeles trainer Kathy Smith, author of the *Power Walk for Weight Loss* DVD, designed the walking workout. Pilates instructor Lara Hudson, author of the *Prevention Fitness Systems: Slim, Strong & Firm* DVD, designed the strength routine.

Add new challenges. If you can talk easily at a brisk pace, go even faster, climb steps, or increase the incline on the treadmill to ramp up the intensity.

TRIPLE-DECKER WALK

These intervals (see "Your Workout at a Glance" on page 173) let you burn more calories for a longer period of time, which translates to more allover slimming.

Warmup, 3 minutes: Go at an easy pace that allows you to sing.

Level 1, 2 minutes: Stride comfortably but purposefully, not so fast that you can't carry on a conversation.

Level 2, 2 minutes: Bump up your heart rate by climbing a set of stairs or a steep hill.

Level 3, 2 minutes: Challenge yourself with a steeper hill or quicken your pace.

Cooldown, 3 minutes: Walk leisurely enough that you can sing.

Weeks 1 and 4: Repeat each level twice.

Weeks 2 and 5: Repeat each level 3 times.

Weeks 3 and 6: Repeat each level 4 times.

SIX PILATES POWER MOVES

These six exercises are graceful, but they're also intense. Precision is vital to results, so start slowly. Try the main moves first; if they're too strenuous, stick with the easier versions, and try to take it up a notch around week 3 (see "Your Workout at a Glance" on page 173).

"Compared with crunches, most Pilates ab exercises challenge the abdominals to a greater degree," says Michele S. Olson, PhD, a professor of exercise science at Auburn University Montgomery. For an even faster payoff, we paired the moves with an exercise band (available at sporting-goods stores): Research shows that adding extra resistance to strength-training almost triples the benefits. These sessions deliver results similar to those experienced by the Skidmore study subjects: flatter abs in shorter workouts.

THE SCISSOR

Works abs, quadriceps, hamstrings, biceps, and shoulders

MAIN move: Seated on the floor, place the center of the band around the ball of your left foot, grasping one end in each hand. Roll down, with your back on the floor, legs extended, feet flexed. Curl your head, neck, and shoulders up, pressing your belly to your spine. With your upper arms on the floor, bend your elbows, bringing your fists to your chest. Lift your left leg straight up over your hip. Using a rapid, controlled motion, inhale and kick your left leg down, stopping just inches from the floor, while lifting your right leg straight up. Exhale and switch legs. Repeat for a total of 8 reps. Switch the band to your right leg and repeat.

Make it easier: Rest your head and shoulders on the floor.

Make it harder: Grasp the band closer to your foot to increase resistance.

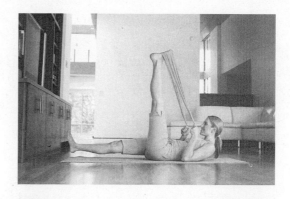

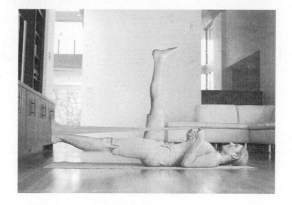

SEATED SIDE TWIST
WITH TRICEPS

Works obliques, back, quadriceps, triceps,
and shoulders

MAIN move: Sit tall with your legs extended and
toes pointed. Bend your left knee, keeping your
foot on the floor, and place the center of the band
under the ball of your foot, holding the band ends
in your left hand. Turn your torso to face your left
knee, wrapping your right hand around your left
knee and squeezing your shoulder blades. Exhale
and lift and extend your left leg to a 45-degree
angle with the floor while straightening and
extending your left arm back at shoulder height
and turning to face your left hand.

KEEPING back erect, inhale as you bend and lower
your leg and arm. Do 8 reps, then switch sides
and repeat.

*Make it easier: Keep both of your feet on the
floor.*

*Make it harder: Instead of holding your knee,
extend your free arm toward your toes at
shoulder height and hold there for the entire
move.*

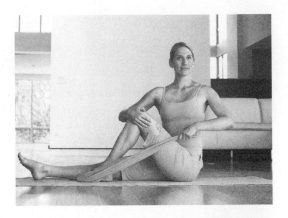

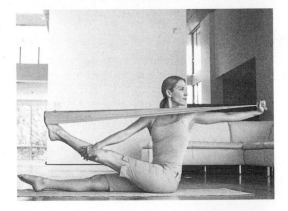

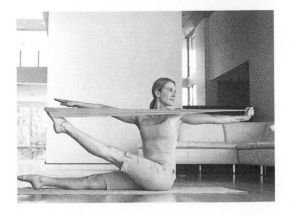

DOUBLE-LEG X

Works abs, back, shoulders, quadriceps,
hips, and biceps

Main move: Seated with your knees bent, place
the band under the balls of both of your feet.
Crisscross the band, holding one end in each
hand, and slowly roll down until your back is on
the floor, keeping your knees bent and bringing
your thighs close to your chest with your feet
flexed. With your upper arms on the floor and
your elbows bent and tucked in, raise your head
and shoulders. That's the start position. Inhale
and straighten your legs out to the sides while
raising your arms out and overhead to form an
X. Keep the movement controlled. Hold for 1
count and return to the start. Repeat for a total
of 8 reps.

*Make it easier: Keep your feet on the floor for
the first 5 reps.*

*Make it harder: Hold the extended position for
5 counts on each rep.*

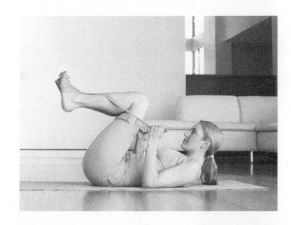

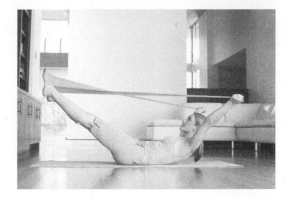

THE BREASTSTROKE

Works back, abs, shoulders, arms, and hips

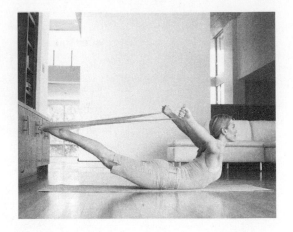

MAIN move: Kneeling with your toes curled under, place the center of the band around the balls of your feet, holding one band end in each hand. Slowly walk out on your hands and lie facedown on the floor, with your feet flexed and your hands on the floor directly beneath your shoulders and your elbows tucked in. Contract your abs and back muscles to lift your head and shoulders gently; exhale and extend your arms forward at shoulder level, lifting your feet at the same time. Circle your arms out to the sides, then in toward your legs and down. Inhaling, circle your wrists to bring your hands back to the floor, under your shoulders, lowering your feet. Do 8 reps.

Make it easier: Hold your chest closer to the floor; don't lift your feet.

Make it harder: As you circle your arms to the sides, open your lifted legs wide and hold for 3 counts before lowering and completing the arm circle.

STARFISH EXTENSION

Works obliques, upper back, outer thighs, and shoulders

MAIN move: Sitting with your knees bent and your feet flat on the floor, place the band around the ball of your right foot, grasping both ends in your right hand. Roll onto your left side with your legs stacked and your knees slightly bent, and rest your right hand on your hip. Aligning your left elbow under your shoulder (left hand forward, fingers spread for support), lift your hips to make a straight line from your knees to your head. Exhale as you lift your right leg, straightening your knee and extending your right arm overhead. Don't sink into your shoulder. Inhale on the release. Complete 4 reps, then switch sides and repeat.

Make it easier: Keep your hips on the floor.

Make it harder: Straighten your bottom leg to form a straight line from your feet to your head.

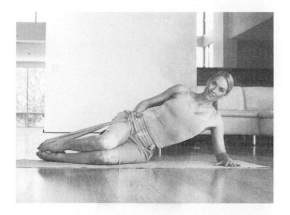

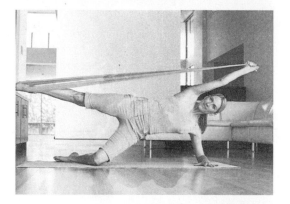

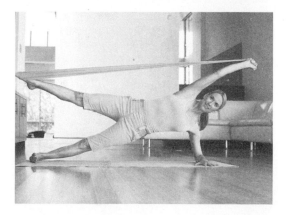

THE HUNDRED

Works abs, triceps, and shoulders

MAIN move: Seated with your knees bent, place the center of the band under your calves, just below your knees. Crisscross the band over your shins and hold one end in each hand, next to your legs. Touching your fingertips to the backs of your thighs, exhale and slowly roll down until your back is on the floor. Lift your knees over your hips, with your lower legs parallel to the floor. Curl your head, neck, and shoulders up, pressing your belly to your spine. Grasping the band in your fists, reach your arms straight out, parallel to the floor. Inhaling, pump your arms rapidly up and down five times. Exhaling, pump arms five times. Repeat for a total of 10 breaths (100 arm pumps).

Make it easier: Rest your head and shoulders on the floor during the exercise.

Make it harder: Grasp the band closer to your legs to increase the resistance.

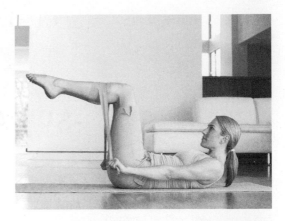

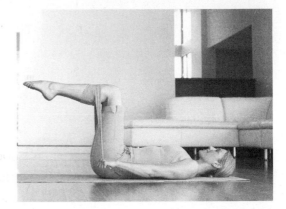

CHAPTER 19

THE NO-SWEAT SLIM DOWN

Ease tension, stand taller, and feel leaner the very first time you do this workout

Imagine a workout that feels as good as a massage and shapes your body like a yoga or Pilates class. That's the payoff of this workout in which you replicate the pressure of a deep-tissue massage by slowly moving your arms, legs, and torso over a small inflatable ball.

"Rolling along the ball loosens up muscles and relieves tension-related pain," says Andrew Pruitt, EdD, director of the Boulder Center for Sports Medicine in Colorado. And supporting your weight and balancing as you roll strengthens and tones your entire body, says Yamuna Zake, author of *The Ultimate Body Rolling Workout*, who designed this 15-minute routine. Even better, you'll feel longer and leaner after just one session.

WORKOUT BASICS

The equipment: You'll need a firm 9-inch ball, such as Yamuna's Body Rolling Ball. Balls come in two degrees of firmness: a softer yellow ball (perfect for beginners) or a harder red ball (for a deeper massage). Balls are sold (pump not included) at www.yamunabodyrolling.com.

The plan: Do each exercise one time, switching sides as directed. You can safely roll every day (rolling complements any type of physical activity and can be a great workout on its own), but aim for at least two or three workouts a week.

Tip

Move slowly and breathe deeply, allowing your weight to sink into the ball. Apply only as much pressure as is comfortable. As with stretching, some good "hurt" is okay, but nothing should feel truly painful.

HAMSTRING RELEASE

Loosens hamstrings, eases back pain, and strengthens abs

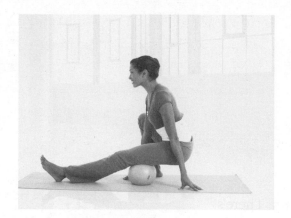

SIT with the ball under your left "sitz" bone (literally the bone you sit on), with your left leg extended, your right leg bent and turned out, and your foot flat on the floor. Lean forward slightly and place your left fingertips on the floor next to your left hip and your right fingertips between your legs for balance. Press off with your fingers and your right foot to pull your buttocks back and roll the ball 3 to 4 inches toward your knee. Take a full breath and roll farther. Continue until the ball rests two-thirds of the way to your knee. Then roll back to the starting position in one smooth movement. Repeat with your opposite leg.

CHEST OPENER

Loosens chest muscles and "deslouches" upper body to improve posture

LIE facedown with the ball at the top of your breastbone, just below your collarbone and above your breasts. Place your forearms on the floor next to the ball, with your fingertips facing forward and your eyes on the floor.

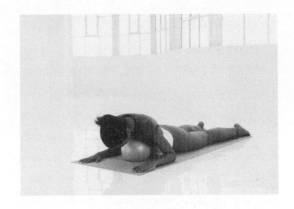

EXTEND your left arm, turn your head to the right, and twist your torso, rolling the ball along your collarbone and under your left arm until it's about two-thirds of the way to your elbow. Roll off the ball and repeat with your right arm.

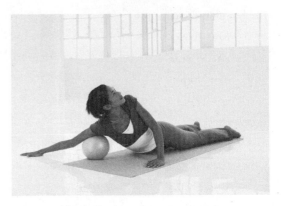

BACK MASSAGER

Relieves back pain, lengthens spine, improves posture, and strengthens core

Sɪᴛ with your legs bent, your feet flat on floor, and the ball under your left sitz bone. Place your hands on the floor slightly behind your body. Drop your buttocks to the floor, rolling the ball from your left sitz bone to the left side of your tailbone. Slowly roll your body along the ball up the left side of your spine. Once the ball is past your lower back, place your left hand on the floor next to you and your right hand behind your head. Keep your head in line with your spine throughout.

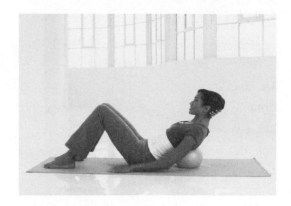

Rᴏʟʟ up the left side of your neck, stopping with your neck and head resting on the ball and your arms at your sides. Pull your shoulders away from your neck as you take a few deep breaths. Then slowly sit up and repeat on your right side.

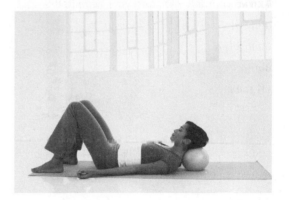

THIGH TONER

Loosens tight hips, relieves some knee pain, and strengthens and tones arms

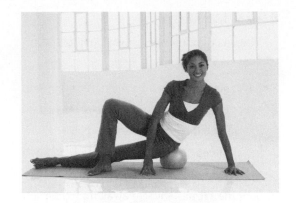

Sit on your left side with the ball beneath your hip. Extend your left leg and cross your right leg in front, placing your right foot flat on the floor. Place your left hand out to the side and your right fingertips in front.

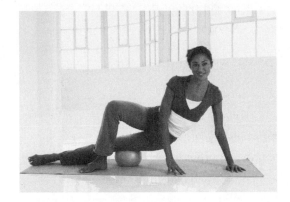

Use your hands to pull your body toward your left hand, rolling the ball down the side of your left leg. About every 2 inches, stop and sink into the ball for about 10 seconds, until the ball is about two-thirds of the way to your knee. Roll back to the starting position in one smooth movement. Switch sides and repeat.

BUTT LIFTER

Loosens tight hips, improves posture, and may ease knee pain

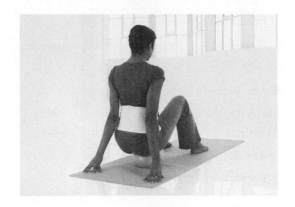

Sit with your legs bent, your feet flat on the floor, and the ball just in front of your left sitz bone where your hamstrings meet the bone. Place your right fingertips on the floor near your right hip. Using your left hand, lift your left buttocks, moving the fat and muscle away from your left sitz bone and sinking deeper into the ball. Place your left fingertips on the floor by your hip.

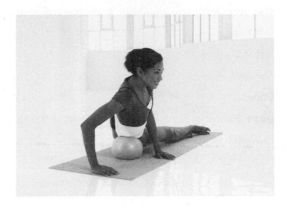

Roll the ball underneath your left sitz bone, moving your right hand to the left side of your body. Slowly drop your left hip toward the floor and extend your left leg as you roll the ball diagonally up to your left hip. Roll back to the starting position and repeat on your opposite side.

CORE STRENGTHENER

Tightens abs and stretches and strengthens back extensors

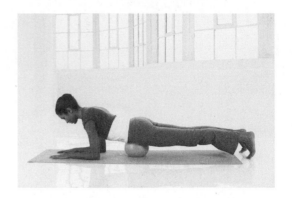

LIE facedown with your pubic bones directly on top of the ball, your upper body propped on your forearms and your legs extended with your knees bent on the floor and your feet flexed. Breathe deeply, sinking into the ball for 30 seconds. Slowly slide your body toward your feet, rolling the ball off your pubic bones and into your lower abdomen. Lift your knees off the floor.

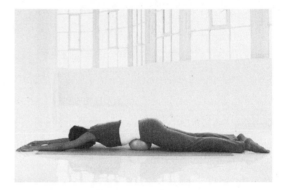

EXTEND your arms overhead, palms down, and point your toes. Take three full breaths, allowing the ball to sink into your abdomen as much as is comfortable, while reaching your arms and legs in opposite directions to stretch your spine and torso. Roll the ball out from under you and relax.

CHAPTER 20

YOGA FOR YOU

Even if you can't reach your toes, you can stand taller, look leaner, and move gracefully with this plan

It's time to forget the idea that yoga is only for the young, the absurdly flexible, or the spiritually inclined. In fact, yoga is a fantastic addition to any fitness plan, no matter your age or ability. And even if you'd never try a scorpion pose, the health benefits of yoga can't be beat. Just one session can temporarily help lower levels of cortisol, a stress hormone linked to a greater risk of heart disease. Research shows that yoga relieves back pain as well as or more effectively than traditional exercises. Still hesitant? You'll also increase strength, get toned, and sleep better.

To get you started, Peggy Cappy, creator of the *Yoga for the Rest of Us* DVD series, designed this easy 15-minute routine that uses a chair to gently increase your flexibility.

"As your body becomes more resilient, your mind will, too," she says. "Everyday stresses, like traffic jams or rude people, won't push your buttons as easily." Perform this routine daily, and you'll be moving with more energy and ease within 2 weeks.

WORKOUT BASICS

The equipment: You'll need comfortable, loose clothing; a mat or carpeted floor; and a sturdy kitchen or dining room chair.

The plan: Do each stretch one time, repeating on the opposite side where instructed. Practice the routine at least three times a week; daily, if possible.

For a challenge: Hold each pose up to 60 seconds.

SHOULDER/WRIST STRETCH

Realigns shoulders that are out of balance from carrying handbags on one side and soothes wrist soreness from too much computer time

SIT on the edge of a chair, keeping your spine erect. Slowly swing your right arm in a large circle, up in front and then down behind you. Start a second circle, but stop when your hand is directly overhead. Keeping your arm up, circle your hand (from your wrist) clockwise two times. Then lower your arm behind you, completing the circle. Do two more arm/wrist circles, and then repeat in the opposite direction, making counterclockwise circles with your wrist. Repeat with your left arm.

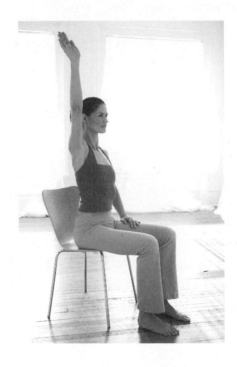

MODIFIED TRIANGLE POSE

Wakes up the whole body by stretching chest, hips, torso, legs, and arms

Stand with a chair seat facing you. Separate your legs about 3 feet, with your left foot under the chair and your toes pointing to the left. Turn your right foot slightly to the left and align the arch of your right foot with the heel of your left. Keep your legs straight. Contract your legs as if hugging muscles to bones. Lengthen your spine and extend your arms out to the sides at shoulder level, palms down.

Keeping your back tall, gently push your hips to the right as you lean to the left, bending at your left hip and placing your left hand on the chair seat. Stretch your right hand toward the ceiling, looking up. Pull your shoulder up and back to keep your torso facing forward. To increase the side stretch, lower your right arm so it extends at a diagonal. Hold for 20 to 30 seconds. Relax and repeat on your right side. As you become more flexible, bend your elbow until your forearm rests on the chair.

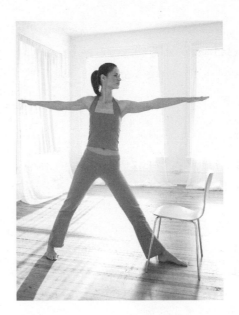

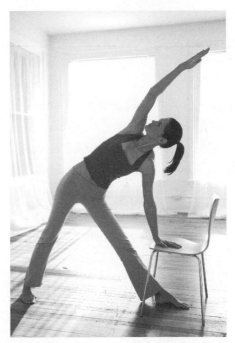

CALF STRETCH

Relieves achy calves, tight Achilles, and cramped toes caused by wearing high heels

START on all fours with your hands beneath your shoulders and your knees beneath your hips. Bring your left knee to your chest, then extend your leg behind you, placing your toes on the floor. Shift your left foot forward an inch, then press your left heel back as though trying to touch it to the floor (it won't actually reach). Hold for 20 seconds. Return to all fours. Repeat with your right leg.

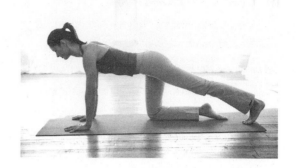

WIDE-LEGGED FORWARD BEND

Stretches lower back, backs of legs, and inner thighs

STAND about 2 feet in front of a chair, with your feet as wide as comfortable. Turn your toes slightly inward and contract your leg muscles, keeping your legs straight. Don't lock your knees. Bend forward from your hips, keeping your back straight. Place your hands on the seat or back of the chair. Keep your head in line with your spine. Hold for 20 to 30 seconds, imagining the space between each vertebra of your spine expanding. As you become more flexible, bend your elbows until your forearms rest on the chair.

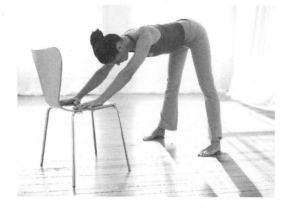

HALF-BOW POSE

Loosens the fronts of thighs, which get tight from too much sitting

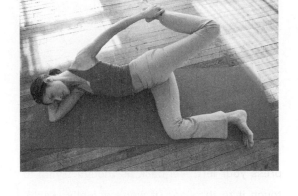

Lie on your right side with your head on your right arm. Pull your knees up until your thighs form a right angle with your torso. Extend your left leg in a line with your upper body. Point, then flex your foot. Hold for 5 to 10 seconds, then relax. Bend your left knee and grab your ankle (or pant leg) with your left hand. Gently pull your foot behind you so you feel a stretch along the front of your thigh. Hold for 20 to 30 seconds, then release your leg. Roll over and repeat with your right leg.

TWIST

Increases back flexibility, so you'll twist more easily the next time you have to parallel park

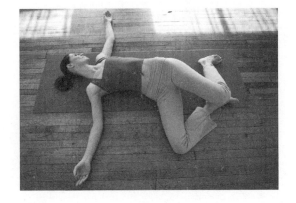

Lying on your back with your arms out to your sides, bend your knees and place your feet hip-width apart and about a foot away from your buttocks. Keeping your shoulders on the floor, slowly drop your knees to the right side as you turn your head to the left. Let your feet roll naturally, and lower your knees as far as comfortably possible. You should feel a stretch along your left side. Hold for 20 to 30 seconds. Return to the starting position and repeat to your opposite side.

MEDICAL BREAKTHROUGHS

Want the latest exercise news? Look no further!

DON'T CHEAT YOURSELF

If you're at risk for diabetes, it's more important than ever not to skip a workout. That's because the insulin efficiency of your muscles decreases after just 2 days of inactivity, according to researchers at the University of Missouri–Columbia. A drop in insulin efficiency can increase your chances of developing diabetes, high blood pressure, and heart disease.

After rest, receptors on muscle cells "become less efficient at signaling the amount of insulin bound to them," and less glucose is taken into your muscles for energy, says study author Frank Booth, PhD, a professor of biomedical sciences. That leaves more glucose to wreak havoc in the rest of your body.

Dr. Booth suggests physical activity most days of the week (walking is good), especially if type 2 diabetes runs in your family.

CRUSH METABOLIC SYNDROME

Slash your risk of diabetes and heart disease by not slacking off on either your diet or exercise program. A Norwegian study of 137 men found that dieting plus exercise is best at reversing metabolic syndrome, a group of symptoms that includes high triglycerides and elevated blood sugar. Sixty-seven percent of men who used the combo—cutting calories and doing 3 hours of cardio per week—were cured of metabolic syndrome in 1 year. Only 23 percent of men who simply exercised and 35 percent who just dieted alleviated their symptoms.

"Exercise and diet impact metabolic syndrome through different mechanisms, so they have an additive effect," says study author Sigmund Anderssen, PhD.

BURN CALORIES, LIVE LONGER

If the treadmill's not your thing, no problem. Two new studies indicate that even mundane activities such as doing chores can tack on years to your life.

The first study, from the National Institute on Aging, followed 302 healthy seniors for 6 years. The most active burned 2,611 calories daily, compared with just 1,766 for the least active group, and the constant movers were 70 percent more likely to be alive at the study's end. The researchers found that for every 287 additional calories the seniors expended each day, their mortality risk dropped 30 percent. The energy difference came from everyday busywork such as cleaning, gardening, and climbing stairs.

In the second study, scientists from the University of Heidelberg in Germany tracked 791 people from their twenties into their senior years and discovered that those who became more active in their forties cut their risk of heart disease by nearly the same amount as those who had maintained a lifetime of activity.

How many calories do you burn in your home "gym"?

ACTIVITY	CALORIES BURNED IN 30 MINUTES*
Raking	146
Climbing stairs	136
Playing with children	136
Washing the dog	119
Sweeping indoors	112
Washing the car	102
Cleaning the garage	102
Washing dishes	78
Making the bed	68

*Based on a 150-pound person.

WALK TO MANAGE YOUR MIDDLE

Research clearly shows that, after age 20, Americans typically gain 10 or more pounds per decade. But it doesn't have to be that way: A new University of Pittsburgh study of 209 middle-aged adults found that walking 30 to 60 minutes a day, five times a week, and maintaining a diet full of fruits and vegetables can help you shed 7 pounds over 1 1/2 years— no dieting required.

SWING YOURSELF SLIM

Those *Dancing with the Stars* contestants aren't just taking one last leap at fame. Well, maybe they are, but they're also getting into seriously good shape.

Mexican researchers tracked 39 people with heart disease who exercised for 30 minutes a day, 5 days a week, for a month. Half the group performed a fast-paced ballroom routine choreographed by a professional dancer, while the rest cycled on stationary bikes. The dancers increased their heart and lung capacity by 28 percent; the cycling group got a 31 percent boost. Experts say it is the quick, uninterrupted movement of up-tempo ballroom dancing that gets your heart pumping.

Add some spice to your workout with lessons at a studio like Arthur Murray (www.arthurmurray.com), or hoof it at home with a DVD. Here are some good choices.

Ballroom Dancing Basics: Learn six fundamental steps you can link together to cut a rug. Close-up shots of the instructors' feet make it easy to mimic their moves.

Ballroom Dancing Made Easy! Examples of proper hand positions and step-by-step footwork instructions help make the steps seem like second nature.

Learn to Dance with John and Charlotte: These *Dancing with the Stars* fan favorites give distinct instructions for both male and female partners, making it simpler to focus on details key to your moves.

SPOT THIS

Hallelujah: Researchers have finally found a workout that may spot reduce. Australian scientists divided 30 women into two groups: Everyone cycled three times a week, but one group rode for 40 minutes at a steady pace, and the other for 20 minutes, alternating 8 seconds of sprinting with 12 seconds of light pedaling. After 15 weeks, the sprinters had lost three times as much body fat as the others—including thigh and core flab, which the rest didn't.

Intermittent sprinting may create a fat-burning response within the exercising muscles, says lead researcher Ethlyn Gail Trapp, PhD. "It seems likely you could stimulate a similar response rowing or running."

To fix your jiggly bits, Trapp suggests trying the 8-second sprints and 12-second slowdowns with any activity targeting your problem areas.

GET OFF THE COUCH!

Sure, sitting on your duff can tip the scale upward. But inactivity also makes losing weight even harder, according to a study in the journal *Diabetes Care*.

Australian researchers measured the blood sugar (glucose) of 4,576 women and found that their levels rose for every hour they spent watching TV.

Extra glucose ends up as fat, explains lead researcher David Dunstan, PhD, of the International Diabetes Institute in Melbourne. And added pounds do more damage by making it tougher for insulin to take extra glucose out of the bloodstream. So go easy on channel surfing: Dunstan's team suggests limiting tube time to 2 hours a day.

WEAR YOUR WALKING SHOES

When you're too swamped to hit the gym, just put on your walking shoes in the a.m. According to an Indiana University study, a few short walks per day can keep you fitter than one sustained workout.

Researchers asked 20 people with borderline high blood pressure to walk on a treadmill at $2^1/_2$ to 4 mph for 40 minutes. On a different day, the subjects walked on the treadmill for four 10-minute periods over the course of $3^1/_2$ hours. The exercisers' blood pressure dropped significantly in each case, but the effect lasted 11 hours when they broke up the workout and 7 hours when they walked continuously.

"Blood pressure is reduced progressively after each short bout of exercise," explains study author Saejong Park, PhD. So when you don't have time for a sweaty run, stay healthy by fitting a few walking breaks into your day.

Success Story

The Weight Rolled Right Off

Barbara Dolan, 43, in Oak Park, Illinois, started skating and found new energy—and a flatter belly!

Barbara had always been slender, and regular dance classes as a young adult helped her stay that way. But in 1999, after her yearlong struggle to get pregnant, the weight piled on right up until she gave birth to her first son. Although the majority of the 40 pounds Barbara gained during pregnancy was healthy, about 13 were over the line—and she never lost them.

During Barbara's second pregnancy 3 years later, she gained 40 again—and kept 20. But as an exhausted mother of two, she simply accepted her 175-pound frame. She was fat; that was that.

Barbara's Call to Action

One day at the playground, Barbara looked around at the other moms and realized that in trying to nurture their families, they'd treated their own bodies with enormous disregard. All around Barbara, she saw cushy bellies, "muffin tops," and back fat. That can't be me, she thought. And yet it was.

Then and there, Barbara decided it was time to change. She didn't want to have to wear "mom jeans"—she wanted to feel sexy again.

Learning How to Get Healthy

Barbara tried Weight Watchers for 3 months, but she found the weigh-ins humiliating, so she switched to the online program. It was just what she needed: Logging in everything she ate made her think of calories in real-world terms. If she had the grilled-cheese crust from her son's plate, she'd forgo wine with dinner to stay within her daily Points range.

To supplement Barbara's online motivation, she asked her husband to take a monthly snapshot of her in a bikini. In each subsequent photo, she looked better than before—and that kept her going! It took 5 months, but she finally met her goal: 142 pounds.

Setting New and Improved Goals

Filled with pride, Barbara had a photographer friend take her portrait. But when she saw the image, she realized she had much more to accomplish. Sure she was smaller, but she was soft all over. The back fat was still there.

So Barbara signed up for Pilates—and got results within a couple of weeks. Her back was stronger and her stomach was toned, but 6 months later, she was no longer enjoying the class. That's when she heard about the Windy City Rollers, Chicago's first all-girl, flat-track roller derby league. Barbara immediately joined.

The three-times-a-week practices were brutal. The women skated, jogged, did calisthenics, and strength-trained—rain or shine. When Barbara started, she'd be wiped after a 20-yard sprint, but soon, she was outskating opposing team members. What a core workout! It took about 6 weeks to notice her tighter tummy, butt, and legs, but the excitement kept her going.

Barbara dropped from a size 16 to a 6 and then lost an additional 7 pounds. Last May, after about 2 years of derby, she hung up her skates. (She began to worry about injury.) But the resolve she got from the sport stays with her. Without it, she wouldn't have had the guts to take on her next challenge: running for public office.

Part V

STRESS LESS

CHAPTER 21

CALM AMID CHAOS

Writer Denise Foley knew that
meditation could help lower her blood
pressure, improve sleep, amp up energy,
and even beat depression. Here's how she
found the alone time to do it

On my first day of meditating at home, I was lying on the floor, trying to focus on my breath. I was also trying to gently push away the intrusive thoughts that were rampaging through my mind like a willful 2-year-old who is being told no.

But my house was filled with family and dogs, and there was a ball game blasting on the TV downstairs. The thoughts I was trying to evict were starting to sound hysterical.

Then I heard it—the clack-clack-clack of dog claws on the hardwood floor. Snuffle, snuffle, snuffle. Buster, our Tibetan spaniel, was inspecting me like a search-and-rescue dog looking for signs of life. Why hadn't I closed the door?

There's a good reason you never see pictures of gurus posing with their families and pets. Can't anybody get a little inner peace around here?

A SKEPTIC IN THE LAND OF ZEN

I'd been assigned to take a meditation class and write about it. The idea wasn't just that it might give me, to borrow a *Seinfeld* catchphrase, "serenity now." The aim was to see whether it could actually fix some of my health issues, such as persistent high blood pressure. Over the past 30 years, studies have found that regular meditation can indeed lower blood pressure—and reduce pain, ease depression, cut anxiety, boost alertness, even make you smarter.

But I expected nothing more than to catch a couple of z's. I'd always found the idea of meditating a little off-putting. Many years ago, I bought a copy of *Full Catastrophe Living* by Jon Kabat-Zinn, PhD, the University of Massachusetts researcher who transformed an ancient Buddhist style of meditation known as mindfulness into something more scientific. The technique is deceptively simple: While focusing on your breathing, you observe your thoughts and sensations but don't attach any emotion to them. When you do that, studies have shown, your heart rate and breathing slow, your metabolism decreases, and your muscles relax, which, over time, can help heal the eroding effect of stress on your body.

When Dr. Kabat-Zinn taught this skill to patients with everything from heart disease to psoriasis, they experienced less stress, anxiety, and pain. They even saw some of their physical symptoms disappear.

I was impressed but not persuaded. Dr. Kabat-Zinn said we should "be in the moment" instead of obsessively reliving the past or anxiously anticipating the future. But I didn't see the payoff. I thought my best bet for happiness was to not be in some of my moments.

I'd been living with the reverberations of the proverbial unhappy childhood (death, boarding school, and parental mental illness are involved), which left me grappling with low-grade depression and a fight-or-flight switch stuck in the on position. What failed to kill me only made me stronger, I figured, but I still

(continued on page 206)

The Payoff of Inner Peace

Sure, nirvana is nice. But here's what else meditation can give you.

A healthier heart: Patients at Cedars-Sinai Medical Center in Los Angeles were able to lower their blood pressure, blood sugar, and insulin—the triumvirate that is primarily responsible for metabolic syndrome, a leading cause of diabetes and heart disease—by practicing Transcendental Meditation, the form associated with a mantra.

Increased alertness: University of Kentucky researchers found that sleepy people who meditated for 40 minutes did better on a test of mental quickness—pressing a button as soon as an image popped up on a computer screen—than people who'd taken a 40-minute nap.

Better sleep: Studies show that meditation can also help you sleep. One Harvard study found that the brain waves of people who are meditating are similar to those seen as people nod off.

More brainpower: Using sophisticated scans, researchers from Harvard, Yale, and elsewhere discovered that experienced meditators had increased thickness in the parts of the brain that deal with attention and processing sensory input—a thicker thinking cap, in other words.

Less bingeing: Mindfulness can help binge eaters recognize when they want to overeat and lower the odds they'll do so. A study done at Indiana State University found that obese women who practiced mindfulness meditation had an average of four fewer binge-eating episodes per week than before they took up the practice.

Happiness: When he scanned the brains of experienced Buddhist practitioners, Richard Davidson, PhD, of the University of Wisconsin–Madison, found their left prefrontal cortexes—the area of the brain responsible in large part for happiness and pleasure—lit up even when they weren't meditating.

needed to take two medications to keep my blood pressure down.

Besides, there was a second stumbling block on the road to bliss: the "find a quiet place where you won't be disturbed for 20 minutes" requirement. Where is that place? I have a husband, a son, and a writing career that involves multiple deadlines, a long-term relationship with the FedEx guy, and 2,645 e-mails. Meditation master Jack Kornfield, PhD, once wrote a book called *After the Ecstasy, the Laundry.* If meditation were to work for me, I'd have to have my ecstasy while doing the laundry.

THE JOURNEY BEGINS

Then I met Diane Reibel, PhD, who teaches Dr. Kabat-Zinn's 8-week Mindfulness-Based Stress Reduction course, or MBSR, at the Jefferson Myrna Brind Center for Integrative Medicine at Thomas Jefferson University in Philadelphia, where she is director of the Mindfulness-Based Stress Reduction Program.

I liked the fact that she was a scientist whose studies on meditation are often cited in other research. And Dr. Reibel was up for an experiment. She was willing to let me bring to class students with specific problems—heart disease, hypertension, eating disorders, anxiety, depression, and lots and lots of stress—to see how meditation worked for them. To chart our progress, we agreed to take assessment tests before the first class and at the end of our last session that were designed to show whether we were depressed, anxious, or in pain and how our emotions were affecting us physically.

Insomnia was one reason Ann Michael joined our group. A poet, essayist, and college professor, Ann, then 47, said that worries made her both exhausted and unable to sleep. "Some days I feel as though I could sleep for 18 hours, and yet I often wake up in the middle of the night," she said.

Ginny Palmer, also a college professor, was 45 when she found out 5 years ago that her "chronic heartburn" was an almost complete blockage of the left anterior descending coronary artery, known as the widow maker. She had a stent—a wire mesh tube—inserted to keep the artery propped open. She started carrying nitroglycerin and low-dose aspirin with her everywhere. "I live with the fear that every time I have an ache or a pain, my arteries could be closing again," she said.

My five other classmates ran the gamut: They were young and old, financially well off and struggling. They hoped meditation would help with headaches, backaches, even post-traumatic stress following a heart attack (three of the women had heart disease).

Jenna Franceski, a then-32-year-old law student, said she's "always had 'food issues.'" Over the past few years, her weight has cycled up and down. "I've always thought meditation was the way to go, but I can't seem to quiet my mind," admitted Jenna, a fast-talking, funny woman whose energy level would make even Katie Couric look depressed. "When I've tried, I've usually fallen asleep."

DAY 1: LEARNING TO BREATHE

Reibel redesigned the MBSR blueprint so that our class of eight met in person only twice: first for a full-day workshop and then for a half-day meeting at the end of the course. The rest of the time we phoned it in, meditating via conference call every Sunday night. During the week, we used guided-meditation CDs for 20 minutes a day.

It was damned noisy in the classroom at Jefferson where we had our first workshop—car horns, police sirens, and jackhammers intruded from the street below. But that was nothing compared with the chaos that flooded my brain seconds after I tried to focus on my breathing, which is the centering practice at the heart of mindfulness. It's supposed to be a way to clear and calm your mind, but my mind was anything but clear and calm. In fact, the cacophony was deafening. First, anxiety: I have five deadlines in the next 6 weeks. I'm never going to make them. Next, recriminations: You shouldn't have taken on more than you could do. Fear marched in. What if no one ever wants me to write for them again?

Then the others arrived: judgments, fantasies, to-do lists, hopes, regrets, crazy stuff out of left field. What's that smell? I should put some pepper on those foamflowers—the rabbits have been nibbling off the blossoms. God, I have so much to do. I should be cleaning the house; it's starting to look like a hovel. Is everyone else having some kind of enlightenment, or am I the only one who can't stop thinking about rabbits and dust bunnies? I need to exercise more. I'll start tomorrow. . . .

Interested in Trying Meditation?

Here are some easy ways to begin.

Read more about it. For a good general overview, try *Meditation for Dummies*, by Stephan Bodian, former editor-in-chief of *Yoga Journal*. It's a concise guide to the various forms, with dozens of self-guided meditations. Or read *Full Catastrophe Living*, by Jon Kabat-Zinn, PhD, to learn about mindfulness meditation and the Mindfulness-Based Stress Reduction (MBSR) program I took.

Pick your path. There are many widely practiced forms of meditation, including mindfulness, Transcendental Meditation (TM), and various spirituality-based practices (for example, Hindu, Christian, Jewish, Tibetan Buddhist). Your choice may be based on your religious beliefs, the proximity of a class, the availability of a book or tape, the time involved, or the cost. Some classes ask for donations, while others have a fee: TM costs $2,500 and is taught over 4 days; an MBSR class, taught over 8 weeks, runs $400 to $550. Dr. Kabat-Zinn's four-CD series of guided meditations is $30—go to www.mindfulnesstapes.com/series1.html.

If that kind of chatter went on in my brain all the time, no wonder I often found myself struggling to put one word in front of the other. I was spending an inordinate amount of energy on mental time travel, toggling between what happened in the past and what I think might happen in the future. And I was way too in touch with my inner critic. Everything that crossed my mind got a thumbs-up or a thumbs-down.

And it hit me. This was why I needed to be in the present moment. The perpetual mental struggle to reconcile the past and control the future was futile, not to mention exhausting.

"Just try to pay attention to your breathing for one full cycle of inhaling and exhaling," Dr. Reibel urged. But before I even began to let my breath out, the thoughts were back, and they'd brought their friends. Once more, I showed them the door.

"Be aware of what you're feeling and

accept what is happening," Dr. Reibel told us. "Let go of judgments and struggle, and be exactly who you are."

WEEKS 1 TO 2: CLEARING THE MIND

Meditation turned out to be like algebra class: I thought I understood it while I was there, but as soon as I was gone, I wanted the number for the homework hotline.

It seemed so simple: You just have to sit undisturbed for 20 minutes each day, which I was willing to insist on and my family was willing to grant, for this 8-week period. You close your eyes and focus on your breath—how your stomach rises when you inhale and falls when you exhale. If you want, you can repeat a word or phrase, either meaningless (a mantra such as *om*) or significant (*peace, love, God*). When other thoughts arise, you gently nudge them away and refocus on your breath or your mantra.

But even with the guided meditation CDs, where a voice talks you through the process, I couldn't start to put a damper on my thoughts until 15 minutes into my 20-minute sessions. I wasn't alone; all of us were having trouble. During our first conference call, Dr. Reibel told us that was perfectly normal. "Just because you have thousands of thoughts doesn't mean you're not meditating," she said. "Just say, 'It's a thought,' then let it go."

Some us of were struggling with more than the difficulty of quieting our minds. As we took turns reporting on our progress, Jean Safran, who'd had a major heart attack 4 years ago in her late fifties, told us she'd canceled a planned vacation in Mexico. Instead, she was heading to Chicago to put her mother in hospice. "I'm meditating every morning and night," she said. She didn't think she could manage without it, but even so, she sounded desperate.

WEEKS 3 TO 5: A SURPRISING CHANGE

I landed a new assignment—one that meant I needed to travel 70 miles every day, making it almost impossible to do a daily 20-minute formal meditation practice. So I turned to what's known in the meditation world as informal practice. At every stoplight in my $2^1/_2$-hour commute, I focused on my breathing. Periodically, I did a "check-in": I stopped and paid attention to how I was feeling and what I was doing. When I had a break, I took a mindful walk on a nearby trail. At home, I even did mindful weeding and clothes folding.

And I noticed a change: My memory was better. I could recall each clump of daffodils I passed. I realized I hadn't lost my keys in a while.

Then something completely unexpected happened. At a routine visit to the doctor, I had to ask the nurse to take my blood pressure twice because I didn't believe it the first time: My reading had dropped 14 points. It wasn't enough for me to give up any meds, but it was significant.

During the next Sunday session, Ginny, the woman with the stent in her artery, announced that her blood pressure had dropped, too—so precipitously that she'd felt dizzy and light-headed. "My doctor told me to cut back on one of my blood pressure medicines," she said. "And if the dizziness continues, I'm supposed to stop taking it altogether."

Ann was also seeing a difference: She was still worried, but she was sleeping better. "Meditation has helped me be more patient with the kids," she added. "They say I'm spacey, but that's better than being the harpy mom screaming at them."

Jenna was falling asleep, too—but during the meditations. "I'm determined to get through it at least once!" she said.

WEEKS 6 TO 8: THE HABIT TAKES HOLD

My meditation sessions were starting to feel important: I was still fitting them into nooks and crannies during my commute, but if I missed one, I'd quickly feel overwhelmed again. I was beginning to think that I'd been wrong to dread being "in the moment"—that the struggle to avoid pain is what actually prolongs it. Meditation doesn't change what happens to you, but it helps change your response. Like the thoughts you gently let go, you realize that life's difficulties, too, will pass.

• • •

"Mindfulness allows you to manage everything more gracefully," Dr. Reibel told me one afternoon as we had lunch at an outdoor café. She should know. Two years ago, she was diagnosed with breast cancer. Her doctor pulled no punches: "He said, 'Diane, the next year will be total hell, but after that you'll get your life back.'" She thought it over and said, "No way. I'm not going to wait. This is my life. I'm going to live it fully, with everything that comes."

Mindfulness has limits, though: You manage with grace; you're not bullet-proof. "I was angry at times," she admitted. "I was scared all the time. And I was in physical pain. But I didn't shut down my emotions."

The old me would have preferred being in a coma for the duration. I said, "That's exactly the kind of moment I never wanted to be in. Don't you wish you didn't have to face it?"

She smiled. "But you have to, if that's what life brings you. The universe isn't here to address our wishes. I look at how I handle life now, compared with before I meditated—I'm not as stressed or afraid. Stress comes from trying to fit life into the box we want it to be in rather than accepting it the way it comes. You might as well live closer to the truth. That's what mindfulness allows you to do."

SERENITY NOW— SORT OF

I've been living closer to the truth for a few months now. Over time, my daily meditations helped me regard what was happening in any moment with curiosity and kindness, without the mindless chatter and instant evaluation that used to whip me into a frenzy. My 19-year-old son was flunking calculus. I resisted the urge to "help" and let him handle it on his own. (He wisely dropped the course.) My deadlines went back to being simply dates; I reminded myself I'd never missed one in my life. My blood pressure stayed down.

Most of my classmates had similar life-changing experiences. Ann dropped her daily meditation practice for a time but found herself waking up again at night. "I went right back to it," she said. She also suspects that meditation pumped up her immune system: For the first time in years, a bout of strep throat didn't turn into bronchitis.

Ginny stopped taking one of her blood pressure medicines. Her BP hovers around 110/70—perfect.

After her mother died, Jean faced other major life events: She was injured at work, a new grandchild was born, and her nest emptied out when her youngest daughter graduated from college. She met it all with uncharacteristic composure. "Meditation kept me in the moment," she said. "It made me realize that no matter what is happening, you can have peace here and now."

Jenna never got over her sleep problem—and was still struggling with her weight obsession when our course ended—but she continued to give herself frequent check-ins during the day, focusing on her breathing, quieting her mind. "It only works for a few seconds, but that's a few seconds more than before," she said.

The questionnaires we filled out before and after the 8-week session showed the strides we made as a class. Our anxiety scores fell 53 percent. Our depression scores dropped by an astonishing 75 percent. And most important for me, I found that you can have ecstasy while doing the laundry. Meditation will always be catch-as-catch-can for me, but even an imperfect practice works. And I never feel guilty if I can't spend 20 minutes meditating in some quiet place where I won't be disturbed. (I still haven't found that paradise.) Even if I miss a few days or just squeeze in a 10-minute check-in with myself between folding the sheets and the delicates, it's all good. Well, it isn't good or bad. It just is.

CHAPTER 22

REASON TO SMILE

Optimists end up healthier and more successful than the rest of us. But guess what? Now researchers have a cheat sheet that can help you become more positive

If you're a pessimist, you can vault yourself into a worst-case scenario in a nanosecond. You get an invitation to dinner from a new neighbor, and you imagine an awkward meal, followed by a lifetime of mutual dislike right on your own block. New clothes are a torment, lying in wait for a ruinous dab of salad dressing. A trip to one of the most beautiful ski resorts in the country? At best, you'll be miserably cold or break an ankle; at worst, you'll wind up snow-blind.

Negativity may appear to be a great defense mechanism: If you keep your expectations low enough, you won't be crushed when things don't work out. But new research has revealed that the tendency to be a wet blanket in just about any situation—a trait the experts call dispositional pessimism— doesn't merely ruin a good time and prevent you from making friends. It seems that it's a bad strategy by about every measure.

Optimists, it turns out, do better in most avenues of life, whether it's work, school, sports, or relationships. They get depressed less often than pessimists do, make more money, and have happier marriages.

And not only in the short run. There's evidence that optimists live longer, too. A 9-year study of cardiovascular health in more than 900 men and women in the Netherlands found that pessimists not only die sooner of heart disease than optimists, but they also die sooner of just about everything. It's enough to drive a pessimist crazy—and sure enough, pessimism has been linked to higher odds of developing dementia.

Fortunately, a grim outlook doesn't have to be permanent. Leading researchers say that optimism and pessimism are two ends of a continuum, with about 80 percent of the US population scattered from mildly to relentlessly optimistic. But research reveals that if you're hunkered down on the other end, you can slide on over—or at least get some of the benefits that usually cluster on the optimistic side of the scale, says Suzanne Segerstrom, PhD, an optimism researcher at the University of Kentucky and author of *Breaking Murphy's Law*. It takes only a few changes. They're small, gradual—and not what you'd expect.

DON'T TRY TO BE HAPPY

In one of Dr. Segerstrom's favorite studies, researchers asked a group of people to use a beautiful piece of classical music to raise their moods, while telling other volunteers simply to listen to the symphony. The result: The concert didn't help those who were focused on lifting their spirits, but the others wound up feeling much better.

"To truly be happy, you have to stop trying," says Dr. Segerstrom. Even monitoring yourself—Am I feeling better yet?—gets in the way, studies show. Instead, aim to be engaged. "Engagement bypasses pessimism," she says. One reason: When you're fully involved in something, it can distract you from a pessimist's favorite pastime—rumination. (That's what psychologists call the destructive pattern of obsessing endlessly over problems or concerns.) When you're ruminating, it's not just a bad day—it's always a bad day, and a bad life, and you're a bad person. The habit will blow up even a minor problem to billboard size. It takes up so much bandwidth, who has room to focus on a solution? It's no surprise that optimists accomplish more than pessimists.

Attitude adjustment: Find quick distractions you can use when you realize you're stuck on the same negative thought, suggests Segerstrom. Try activities that demand your full attention: Go to a yoga class (or a kickboxing or aerobics class, where you have to commit fully to avoid falling on your face). At the office, try calling a friend or switching on some absorbing music.

IMAGINE THAT IT'S THE END OF THE WORLD

Ruminating is just one road to pessimism. Another habit that dims your outlook: a process called catastrophizing, mentally rewriting grim possibilities until they become true doomsday scenarios. A simple cough turns into pneumonia (and not the kind you recover from either). One missed deadline is the first step in a fast trip to permanent unemployment.

This rumination/catastrophization combo packs a terrible one-two punch: Those worst-case scenarios may be absurd, but playing them over and over makes them seem not only logical but inevitable. And it sucks all the joy out of life.

Attitude adjustment: Exaggerate those scenarios to the point of comic hilarity, says Karen Reivich, PhD, codirector of the Penn Resiliency Project at the University of Pennsylvania and coauthor of *The Resilience Factor*. "At some point you think, 'Oh, come on, now. Am I really going to be living beneath an underpass in a refrigerator box because I'm a day late on a project?'"

Don't stop with the refrigerator box. Picture yourself trying to trap squirrels for supper—maybe even whipping up some squirrel fondue for the other homeless people you've met under the bridge. Then paint the opposite scenario: Your project makes your company a million dollars! You're promoted to CEO! Finally, write down the outcome that's most likely. Chances are, it won't include the executive suite—or the one under the freeway.

"The beauty of this goofing around is that you feel a bit of power over your thoughts and the situation," Dr. Reivich says. "That sense of control is the antidote to pessimism."

GO AHEAD, BLAME SOMEONE ELSE

Researchers have learned that optimism and pessimism both boil down to little more than an "explanatory" style—a person's distinct way of interpreting life's ups and downs. When a good thing happens, pessimists dismiss it as a fluke; optimists take the credit. When bad things happen, pessimists blame themselves and expect to suffer a long time, while optimists see bad events as having little to do with them and as one time problems that will pass quickly. A pessimist who misses a shot on the tennis court says, "I'm lousy at tennis"; an optimist says, "My opponent has a killer serve."

University of Pennsylvania psychologist Martin E. P. Seligman, PhD, author of *Learned Optimism* and a pioneer of positive psychology, was the first to discover that a person's explanatory style is fairly stable—and that it often explains why pessimists fail when optimists succeed. After all, it's easier to keep practicing your tennis serve if you're sure you'll do fine against someone at your level.

Thanks to the power of their explanatory style, optimists have an easier time even when things go wrong. Optimistic breast cancer patients are just as depressed by bad news as their pessimistic counterparts, researchers have found. But women with an optimistic disposition are more likely to expect their cancer ordeal to have a positive outcome, studies show; not surprisingly, these women report significantly greater emotional well-being during treatment, while pessimists suffer more distress.

The good news: Researchers have found that pessimistic, self-blaming people can learn to come up with alternative explanations for setbacks and move forward to problem solving. However, making a long-term mind-set switch takes continuous effort.

Attitude adjustment: When you catch yourself thinking like a pessimist, reframe the problem so that it's not all your fault. Instead of standing alone at a party thinking, "No one is interested in talking with me—I look pathetic!" try something like "Where's the hostess? I'd never let a newcomer fend for herself without making introductions!"

Of course, a true optimist wouldn't go looking for a scapegoat—and you do have to acknowledge your contribution to a problem if you want to make it better. But it helps to recognize that you're not the problem, even if your behavior could use some tweaking. Finally, set a small, achievable goal: Find that hostess and ask her to introduce you to three people at the party.

TRY, TRY AGAIN

Why do optimists tend to end up with so much to feel good about? Long after pessimists have given up and gone home, optimists keep trying to solve problems. In one study, optimists continued to work on unscrambling an impossible-to-solve anagram 50 to 100 percent longer than pessimists.

There wasn't a lot of payoff for persistence in the anagram exercise (and the pessimists are still thinking, "Suckers!"). But in the real world, studies show that persistence leads to more success in school, a fatter paycheck, and a host of other perks.

In fact, in a study of law students, Dr. Segerstrom found that a person's level of optimism in the first year of law school corresponded with his or her salary 10 years later. The impact wasn't measly: On a 5-point scale, every 1-point increase in optimism translated into a $33,000 bump in annual income.

Attitude adjustment: The quickest way to get yourself into the positive-feedback loop that keeps optimists going strong (hard work leads to success, which leads to more self-confidence and a willingness to work even harder, which leads to . . .) is to act like one. What's more, studies looking at the "fake it till you make it" approach show that it can have a surprisingly strong—and immediate—impact on your emotions.

In research at Wake Forest University, for example, scientists asked a group of 50 students to act like extroverts for 15 minutes in a group discussion, even if they didn't feel like it. The more assertive and energetic the students acted, the happier they were.

What's best about this kind of cognitive behavioral change is that it doesn't even require much faith, Dr. Segerstrom says. "You don't have to believe an antibiotic is going to work for it to work."

The same is true of reaping the benefits of adopting a positive mind-set.

MAKE FRIENDS WITH AN OPTIMIST

If you're not in the mood for playacting, hooking up with an optimist may be the next best strategy. A yearlong study of more than 100 college-age couples from the University of Oregon found that both positive thinkers and their partners have greater satisfaction in their relationships than optimist-free pairs, in part because happy-go-lucky types tend to see their partners as supportive.

"If you are the partner of an optimist, both of you will be more satisfied in the relationship and more constructive in resolving conflicts," says Sanjay Srivastava, PhD, lead researcher on the study. It's not that a rosy worldview is contagious, it's just that you'll feel more positive about the relationship.

Attitude adjustment: Besides "slip-streaming" on your partner's optimism, socialize with cheery friends and bounce ideas off your more positive colleagues; research hints that these kinds of relationships with up-side types can make you feel better, too. And if you happen to be married to a pessimist or are on your own? Your optimistic friends and co-workers are your best sounding board.

CHAPTER 23

THE POWER OF FORGIVENESS

Five steps that get you past your anger—and into a happier, healthier life

Joan Borysenko, PhD, was about 10 when her mother had a fight with her best friend, Selma. Summer days at the Smiths' pool suddenly were a thing of the past; so were the festive Wednesday night poker games at Selma's house. Any mention of the woman Joan had thought of as an aunt—indeed, Selma's very name—was enough to make Joan's mother livid. They didn't reconcile for more than a decade. The grievance that split them apart? An argument over who would pay for a bag of groceries.

Buddha would say that Joan's mother's resentment was like a hot coal: She picked it up to throw it at someone else, but she was the one who got burned. Frederic Luskin, PhD, and Carl Thoresen, PhD, who run the Stanford Forgiveness Project at Stanford University, have shown that a grudge is a gift that keeps on giving—misery, that is. It causes anxiety, depression, anger, paranoia, isolation, insomnia, and physical pain. But by forgiving your transgressor, you take back control of your life, and that brings just as outsized a list of benefits. There are physical pay-offs, such as lower blood pressure; maybe more important, you feel less anger, anxiety, and depression and more self-esteem.

One of the most moving of Luskin's studies was the Stanford–Northern Ireland Hope Project, in which 17 men and women from Northern Ireland, all with family members murdered in the violence there, went to Stanford for forgiveness training. After just a week, these men and women who'd lost parents, children, spouses, and siblings reported a 35 percent decline in headaches, stomachaches, and other symptoms of stress and a 20 percent drop in symptoms of depression.

Most people think forgiveness is a good idea, Luskin says—"until they have something to forgive." That may be because so many of us just don't know where to start. Fortunately, the path has been well marked, and one of the best decisions you can make is to learn how to follow it. Here are five steps to start you on your way.

Understand what forgiveness is—and what it isn't. A lot of people don't want to forgive because they think it's wimpy or that it means they're saying the offender did nothing wrong. It's neither: You can send an offender to jail and forgive him.

People also think forgiveness requires reconciling with the person who mistreated them. It can—but it doesn't have to. Forgiveness isn't really about the offender at all. Instead, it's about letting go of the anger that eats at you—accepting that you were wronged but deciding to move on from your hurt. It's an act of profound self-respect and self-care that takes courage and commitment on your part.

Grieve for what you've lost. Premature forgiveness has been compared with squirting whipped cream over garbage. The result may look good, but the underlying problem remains and will fester. To truly forgive, you must feel your sorrow, and that can take time.

Even after you've decided to let go of your anger, you may feel it flare from time to time. You need to be gentle with yourself, counsels educator Robin Casarjian, founder of the Lionheart Foundation, a national prison rehabilitation program. In time, the memory of what happened will return less often and feel less painful.

Don't wait for an apology. Sometimes the person who hurt you isn't even aware

---

Smart Ways to Really Move On

Take a calming breath. When an upsetting memory arises, use deep breathing or another stress-management technique to allow yourself to feel your emotions without becoming overwhelmed by them.

Change the way you describe yourself. You were badly hurt, but you're also someone who was brave enough to choose to forgive.

Tell it one more time. Acknowledge your hurt to someone you trust, and then stop telling your grievance story once and for all. These stories keep hurt alive and can prevent you from being fully open to the people you need and love.

---

that he's done so. In other cases, he's incapable of understanding or caring. The simple words *I'm sorry* can be healing, but so is deciding that you no longer need to hear them.

Try to understand what drove the offender. Generally speaking, bad behavior is the result of emotional immaturity, a state more to be pitied than judged. For example, studies show that many of the criminals in our federal prisons were abused as children. If your ex-friend betrayed a confidence, what insecurity must have driven her? If your father never showed you love and affection, how damaged must he be?

Empathy can force out corrosive anger and transform your life—and some-times the lives of others. Consider the story of Cheryl Ward, whose husband had been killed and her daughter raped when a gang of teenage boys broke into their home looking for money. Cheryl has a story of radical empathy: Rather than being consumed by her grief and anger, she chose to visit the young men in prison and try to understand what had prompted them to commit such a heinous crime. Developing compassion not only lessened her pain but also led her to become an advocate for inmate rehabilitation.

Celebrate who you have become. In a recent study at the University of Miami, psychologist Michael McCullough, PhD, and his colleagues asked approximately

200 people who'd been hurt by someone to write about either the traumatic aspects of the betrayal or things they'd gained as a consequence, such as becoming less selfish or discovering that they had unexpected strength. Those who wrote about what they'd learned or how they'd grown described feeling less bitter than the others did and were also more likely to forgive.

Life is a school for learning, and some of the lessons are painful ones. We can't avoid being hurt. But we can decide not to let our hurt overshadow the rest of our lives. Choosing to let go and move on doesn't leave you the same as you were before. It brings you greater understanding and maturity and more compassion—toward others, and toward yourself as well.

CHAPTER 24

PEACE AMID STRESS

De-stress your day with these expert tips

We teamed up four worn-out women with the ideal tension-taming experts for 3 weeks. Steal their tips to de-stress your life.

"HEALTH WORRIES KEEP ME UP AT NIGHT"

"I've had six surgeries since I was diagnosed with breast cancer 2 years ago," says Linda Mastaglio, 53. "But I realize I'm lucky to be alive, and being grumpy is disrespectful to myself."

Although Linda has been breast cancer free since fall 2005, she still worries that her disease will return. Her anxiety about the future of her health and her steady stream of work deadlines nag her at bedtime.

We asked Anne Coscarelli, PhD, director of the Ted Mann Family Resource Center at UCLA's Jonsson Comprehensive Cancer Center, to offer Linda help.

Reframe stress. Linda continues to have a lot of appointments, each a 45-minute commute away. To make this time rejuvenating instead of stressful, Dr. Coscarelli suggests listening to audiobooks. When Linda arrives, she should have job-related materials to work on while she is waiting so she can use the time more productively. And before bed each night, Linda should play a relaxation CD. "This will help retrain her brain to cope with stress better," Dr. Coscarelli says.

Set boundaries. When cancer-related worries come to mind, Linda should engage in positive self-talk, telling herself something like "This is a temporary period of stress. I have no reason to believe I'm not healthy." When a random ache or pain crops up, she could try "If this continues for X days, I will call my doctor and schedule a checkup. Until then, I will do my best to function as usual."

Embrace *no*. Linda is a classic "yes-woman." She rarely refuses a tempting work assignment, even though she's often overloaded, so she feels like she's running from deadline to deadline. Before agreeing to any new work, Linda should ask herself, "Is this something I really want and need to take on? Will this mean I have too much work to do?"

The Results

Biggest surprise: "I had no idea a 30-minute relaxation CD could do so much!

From the first night on, the breathing and positive-thinking exercises simply made it easier for me to let go of my worries. I fell asleep faster and woke up less often throughout the night. I also started listening to audiobooks while commuting. I finally got to 'read' *The 7 Habits of Highly Effective People,* which I had long wanted to dive into. Actually accomplishing something while commuting felt great."

Best advice: "A few weeks ago, a sore arm had me scared that my cancer was back and spreading to my bones. Instead of getting carried away, I took Anne's advice and told myself if the pain was still there after 3 days, I'd see a doctor. Because I had a plan, I no longer had this vague threat I needed to worry about. This has truly altered my approach to my health."

Toughest tip: "The advice on saying no was the hardest. While I did ask myself, 'Is this a good idea?' before I said yes, I still said yes 99 percent of the time. I'm not a pushover; I just love what I do. That alone helped me rethink work as a blessing rather than a source of stress.

"At first I was concerned that this makeover would just be one more thing on my to-do list. I was wrong. I feel like these small steps have transformed my life."—Linda

"DOING IT ALL WEARS ME DOWN"

"Between my husband's erratic career and my nonstop work schedule, I couldn't catch my breath," says Terri Slater, 49.

Since Terri's husband left his steady job to go freelance, she's become the primary breadwinner. Her 50-hour workweeks leave little time for anything else.

We tapped Tina B. Tessina, PhD, author of *The Ten Smartest Decisions a Woman Can Make after Forty*, to help Terri out.

Enlist the troops. Terri does most of the housework. She needs to ask her family to pick a minimum of two chores they each can do per week, then hang a list of everyone's duties on the fridge.

Ring in relaxation. To keep her energy up, Terri should set an alarm to remind her to take a stroll (even just a quick one will help) at lunch and again at 3 p.m.

Offer unbiased help. Terri feels tense about her husband's search for work.

She should volunteer her help but assure him she'll keep her negative opinions to herself. It will let her feel more involved.

The Results

Biggest surprise: "I can't believe the difference my twice-daily walks made. Once the alert sounded on my computer, I'd stop whatever I was knee-deep in and take the dog for a stroll. It got my blood flowing and cleared my head. I thought it would be hard to get back into the groove after these breaks, but I was actually more productive. Tina also suggested shaving a bit of time off my workday. I now can do my favorite yoga tape and get in 15 to 30 minutes of exercise before making dinner. It's brilliant."

Best advice: "My family didn't even blink when I asked for help. Before I knew it, I no longer had to worry about picking up dry cleaning, scrubbing the bathroom, or doing laundry. It was a major wake-up call: I do have support; I just had to ask for it."

Toughest tip: "One of my biggest sources of stress—my husband's unstable income—is still a struggle, but I feel like we're on a better path. He even let me help him revamp his résumé, which made us both feel good.

"Simply knowing my family was there for me made a world of difference. I felt so appreciated and respected."—Terri

"MY MOTHER REALLY NEEDS ME"

By this time in her life, Barbara Meltzer, 64, thought she'd be retired and relaxing. Instead, she's running her own company and is the primary caregiver for her elderly mother.

We asked Marion Somers, PhD, former manager of the Professional Geriatric Care Management Certificate Program at Hunter College's Brookdale Center on Aging, for advice.

Delegate tasks. Barbara should allow someone else, like a nurse's aide, to take on at least three tasks a week for her mother. Also, she could reduce the length of her 4-days-a-week, 1- to 3-hour visits. With the time gained, she could do something fun.

Set small goals. To regain control of her unorganized home and high-stress job and feel less overwhelmed, Dr. Somers suggests Barbara set more manageable goals. So instead of thinking, "I need to redo the bedroom," concentrate on organizing one corner on a Saturday afternoon.

Start with calm. Each morning, Barbara needs to earmark 15 minutes to do nothing but meditate, stretch, or take a brisk walk. If "me" time is the first priority of the day, it's less likely to be pushed aside, Somers says.

The Results

Biggest surprise: "Putting aside 15 minutes for myself had a huge impact. My before-breakfast walk really set the tone for the day. I focused on my surroundings and the fresh air—not on everyone else."

Best advice: "I started carving out 15-minute blocks to tackle tasks, such as sorting through piles of papers. Little by little, my apartment, my office, and my life have become significantly less cluttered."

Toughest tip: "I can't bear to let others take care of my mom. Although it means less free time, I actually feel less stressed in the long run if I'm there for her. But I did delegate more at work and was surprised how much more I could accomplish because of it.

"Letting go of my need to do everything at the office has been a revelation.

I feel more relaxed and able to accomplish more things in my life."—Barbara

"MY HUSBAND DOESN'T PITCH IN"

Leigh Devine, 43, hasn't been able to tell her husband that she's unhappy with the imbalance of chores and responsibilities between them.

We introduced Leigh to Darlene Mininni, PhD, author of *The Emotional Toolkit*, to help teach this married mom how good communication can beat stress.

Confess money concerns. Before her baby arrived, Leigh paid one-third of the bills while her husband handled two-thirds. Now that Leigh doesn't have as much time to work, she's not making as much money, so she can't keep up. Having to dip into her savings to pay for expenses is stressing her out. "She needs to sit down with her husband to come up with a new financial plan, and she must be clear that the current setup no longer works for them," Dr. Mininni says.

Speak, don't seethe. Because husbands don't have psychic powers, Leigh should spell out exactly what she needs—whether it's help around the house or an hour alone while he watches the baby—and how his lack of help makes her feel (i.e., overwhelmed, upset, worried).

Build a partnership. They should plan at least one family event each week and put it on a communal calendar. At the same time, Leigh should give her husband a heads-up about a yoga class that she'd like to take regularly, put it on the calendar, and let him care for their daughter while she's exercising. These small steps build trust and respect—and will create a stronger bond between the two of them. And writing events down in black-and-white means these activities are less likely to be pushed aside.

The Results

Biggest surprise: "I thought keeping activities like dinner out with my husband on the calendar would help change him, but it turned out that it changed me, too. I realized that I do have some time in my life for the things I enjoy. We're really trying to do things together more. My husband even arranged for child care during our recent vacation to Florida so we could spend some time reconnecting without having to worry about our daughter."

Best advice: "When I started talking

about our money situation, there were tears on my end. When I really started explaining my feelings, I think my husband finally began to understand how heavily our finances weigh on me. Although we didn't finish our conversation with a concrete plan like I'd hoped, something struck a chord with my husband. He has been paying for more of our joint expenses. I feel that he really heard my money concerns."

Toughest tip: "At first, I didn't feel supported when I asked for more help with child care. I have to say, I was shocked by his original reaction. But once I started putting activities like my yoga class in ink—letting him know I was serious and he'd be watching the baby while I was gone—he began respecting my time a lot more.

"I keep my makeover tips at the ready on my computer so that I can refer to them regularly. I feel so much more confident now in my abilities and in my marriage."—Leigh

MEDICAL BREAKTHROUGHS

Reducing stress is important for your overall heath, as well as for your life with diabetes. Here's the latest research on stress.

RELAX INSTANTLY

A British survey of 2,000 adults reports that 84 percent of people feel instantly relaxed when they're in nature. Of those, 42 percent preferred gazing at the sea, 33 percent picked a stroll in the park, and 14 percent found calm by listening to birds singing.

GET MORE Z'S

You may be snoozing even less than you think. Americans spend about $7 \frac{1}{2}$ hours a night in bed, but that includes awake time. New research published in the *American Journal of Epidemiology* indicates we sleep only about 6 hours. Our time between the sheets is often spent stressing about money or work.

Why pop a pill when you can dress to drift off? Socks may help you fall asleep faster, say Dutch researchers who measured how long it took for eight healthy people to fall asleep on six different occasions, changing what they wore and did prior to lights-out. The only factor that mattered: pulling on a pair of socks. Compared with when they were barefoot, people who wore socks conked out 27 percent faster. "Increases in the temperature of your feet signal neurons in your brain that cause you to fall asleep," says lead author Roy Raymann, PhD. Wait until just before bed; people who warmed their feet early didn't see the same benefit.

HAVE A SPOT OF TEA

Drinking black tea may keep you calm after an upsetting experience, suggests a new report from University College London. Researchers asked 75 adults to drink either real or fake tea four times a day for 6 weeks. Then the study leaders put them through a stressful encounter (volunteers were accused of shoplifting or told they could be laid off, for example). The tea drinkers' cortisol levels remained 20 percent lower than those of people who consumed the faux tea. To reap the same benefits, drink black tea, derived from the evergreen shrub *Camellia sinensis*—not herbal or other varieties. We like Tazo's Awake tea.

E-MAIL A HIGHER POWER

Reaching out to God (even if it's via the Web) may help you cope with illness. Studying an online breast cancer support group, researchers found links between how optimistic patients felt and how often they used words like *pray, faith,* and *God*.

Women who used them the most felt less pessimistic and healthier overall. Sharing their beliefs bolstered their sense of well-being, says Bret Shaw, PhD, who led the University of Wisconsin–Madison study. "They were better able to be positive and find blessings in their lives."

Interestingly, 77 percent of physicians say they're willing to pray with patients.

BUST A GUT

Turns out *Scrubs* is good for your waistline. According to a study in the *International Journal of Obesity*, laughing out loud can help you burn more calories. For 90 minutes, 45 people watched videos that were either funny (*Austin Powers*) or big snooze fests (a show about the English countryside) while scientists measured their heart rate and calorie burn. Laughing out loud increased both numbers by up to 20 percent, compared with watching quietly. So giggle for 15 minutes a day—you could burn as many as 50 calories.

Success Story

She Prayed for Help to Outsmart Diabetes

Something felt terribly wrong when Jacqueline Daniels, 45, from Cincinnati, Ohio, returned to her job as a nursing-home aide last January after surgery. "After 2 days back at work," she recalls, "I felt so weak that I asked one of the nurses to check my blood sugar. [Jacqueline's aunt and uncle both have diabetes.] It was 380." A normal, nonfasting level is 125 milligrams per deciliter (mg/dL) or lower. "They rushed me to the hospital. I found out later I was close to death."

Jacqueline was determined not to end up like the patients with diabetes she cares for: "I've seen them lose limbs, lose their eyesight, and pass away. I never thought it would happen to me, and I didn't know what to do. I cried." Everything she ate seemed to raise her blood sugar.

The turning point: Once she returned to work, she looked for help. "One of the nurses said, 'Eat less. Check your sugar more often. Instead of a whole apple, eat one-fourth and see what happens.'"

Jacqueline prayed with the nursing-home chaplain. "I remembered that little verse, 'God grant me the serenity. . .' That helped me a lot," she says. She also met with a certified diabetes educator—someone trained to help people with diabetes deal with nutrition and lifestyle issues—who worked with her to develop a practical eating and activity plan. Jacqueline left the appointment ready to overhaul not just her own life but also her family's. Later, she joined a University of Cincinnati research study that's looking at the effects of portion control on blood sugar.

"I used to eat a lot of meat—I love pig's feet—and bread. Instead, I started having more salad, chicken, fish, and veggie burgers because of everything I've learned," she says. "We always had sugary soda pop and chips in the house. That

(continued)

Success Story (cont.)

all changed. The kids didn't like it at first. They kicked and screamed. But now they beat me to the refrigerator. They like these healthy foods." In her kitchen: diet drinks, fruits and veggies, lean meats, baked chips, and low-fat popcorn.

"I try to walk for at least 30 minutes a day and make the kids come, too," she adds. "On Saturdays, we walk to my brother's produce stand at Findlay Market, where I sometimes help out. It's a great place to get fruits and vegetables."

Jacqueline now eats seven small meals and snacks per day, up from two or three large meals. She tracks her carbohydrate intake and measures healthy portions with a clever trick: comparing serving sizes to her hand. "A 5-ounce serving of protein is equal to my palm; a cup of pasta is about the size of my fist. It's a system I can take with me anywhere."

The results? "Now I can laugh at diabetes. At work, they call me Miss Diabetical," says Jacqueline, who also stopped smoking. Gone, too, is her quick temper. "I used to whoop and holler and get mad about everything," she says. "But that really kicks my blood sugar up. It isn't easy, but now I try to pray for someone who's making me mad. I just walk away. We're only here on earth for a short moment. I have a lot left to do."

PART VI

AVOID COMPLICATIONS

CHAPTER 25

HEART SMARTS

Drawing upon new research, South Beach Diet cardiologist Arthur Agatston suggests we can detect and prevent heart disease earlier than ever. Reporter Kathleen McAuliffe investigates

Heart disease is our biggest killer, period. Despite our fears of cancer, terrorism, violent crime, and flying, heart problems snuff out some 871,500 lives a year, 36.3 percent of all deaths or 1 of every 2.8 deaths.

To make matters worse, according to the American Diabetes Association, most people with diabetes have risk factors that increase their risk of heart disease and stroke, such as high blood pressure and cholesterol. In fact, more than 65 percent of people with diabetes die from heart disease or stroke. With diabetes, heart attacks occur earlier in life and often result in death.

It doesn't have to be that way, says preventive cardiologist Arthur Agatston, MD, who developed the widely known South Beach Diet. He believes we have the tools in hand right now to stem this epidemic.

"You don't have to have a heart attack," Dr. Agatston insists, and his new book, *The South Beach Heart Program*, is his comprehensive guide to helping make sure Americans don't.

Preventing heart disease is not a recent cause for Dr. Agatston. He developed the South Beach Diet specifically for his high-risk heart patients. And if you've ever had a computer tomography (CT) heart scan, you may have heard your result referred to as the Agatston score: He developed this measure of calcified plaque in arteries, which indicates heart risk—testimony to his contribution to the field.

Dr. Agatston argues that by combining this screening test with other sophisticated new ones, Americans can identify their heart risk years or decades earlier—and with more precision—than ever before. And with targeted prevention involving special drugs and the proper combination of smart eating and exercise, we can wipe out heart disease just as we eradicated polio and rickets.

"At our clinic and at other top heart clinics across the country, our patients almost never have heart attacks," Dr. Agatston says. "We only see one or two a year—and those are primarily in patients who don't take their meds." He makes a persuasive case, but not all cardiologists are on board: The value of these heart-screening tools in saving lives is among the most controversial issues in cardiology today.

I decided the best way to learn about Dr. Agatston's aggressive, proactive approach is to offer myself as a guinea pig. I also bring along a friend, Stacey Berkley Devine, a Miami-based harpist and yoga instructor who knows firsthand the toll of heart disease. Her father died of a heart attack at 49; Stacey recently turned 50.

DAY 1: A MAMMOGRAM FOR THE HEART

On a bright October morning, we arrive at the waiting room of Dr. Agatston's plush new clinic in the heart of South Beach feeling cranky and on edge. Since midnight the day before, we have had to forgo food and coffee for our first screen—a blood test to gauge our fasting levels of glucose, various types of cholesterol, and other markers.

Fortunately for everyone, we are soon ushered in to meet Dr. Agatston. He's a thin, youthful-looking man of 59 with only a sprinkling of gray in his hair. His

Pricing Out the New Tests

Preventive cardiologist Arthur Agatston, MD, recommends these tests to people with one or more of the following risk factors: having diabetes, high blood pressure, or a family history of heart disease; or being overweight or postmenopausal. Most doctors can set up the screens for you. Just remember—these are brand-new tests, not part of a regular blood test, and your insurance may not cover some of them.

TEST	C-REACTIVE PROTEIN	HOMO-CYSTEINE	LIPOPRO-TEIN(A)	ULTRA-SOUND OF CAROTID ARTERY	PLAIN TREAD-MILL STRESS TEST	CT SCAN WITH DYE
Cost	$45	$75	$95	$400	$250	$1,100
What it screens for	Marker of inflammation that may promote the rupture of plaque	Amino acid that increases risk of vascular disease and amplifies bad effects of other risk factors	Independent risk factor for plaque buildup	Thickening of the artery and presence of plaque	Blockages in coronary arteries and overall fitness	Hard plaque, associated with old ruptures, and soft plaque, the source of potential ruptures
High-risk result	>3.0 mg/dL	>10 mg/dL	>30 mg/dL	>0.8 mm and large amount of plaque	Abnormal EKG	More calcified plaque than expected for your age

skin has the rosy glow of someone who exercises regularly.

He greets Stacey and me with a smile: "My aim is to make sure you're as healthy as you appear to be," he says. The standard blood panel and physical miss too many people with significant cardiovascular disease, explains Dr. Agatston: "I'm trying to get a more complete picture of your risk. If you have hidden heart disease, I want to know now, because we can stop further damage to your cardiovascular system."

We fill out questionnaires about our health, fitness, and family history of disease and then offer up our forearms for the blood sample. Then Dr. Agatston lays out a plan for how we will proceed—and it quickly becomes clear how his approach differs from that of almost all other cardiologists. At minimum, he says, he wants us to get a treadmill stress test and ultrasound of the carotid arteries in the neck, which provide the main supply of blood to the brain. Most doctors wouldn't screen at-risk patients for this, let alone apparently healthy women like Stacey and me. Then, depending on the results of our blood work, he might recommend a 64-slice CT scan of the heart.

"What would that tell me?" I ask.

Dr. Agatston shows us CT pictures on a large flat-panel screen mounted on the wall next to his desk. With his pointer, he targets blockages in the major artery of the patient's heart that even our untrained eyes can readily spot.

Better yet, the scan distinguishes between hard plaque—the calcified patches where cholesterol lining the arteries had ruptured and healed over—and more dangerous soft plaque, the source of new, potentially lethal ruptures. "It can catch problems way ahead of any symptoms," he says. "I call this test a mammogram for the heart."

Dr. Agatston runs his pointer over the inside wall of an artery. "See this bump that looks like a pimple? It's called soft plaque. It used to be impossible to see, but now we have this new technology that uses a dye to highlight it. When soft plaque ruptures, if the blood clot that forms around the lesion is large enough, it can impede bloodflow, starving the heart of oxygen. That's what triggers a heart attack."

But then he tells me that, at 51, I'm not yet menopausal, and therefore my risk isn't high enough to warrant the scan. Of course, now I want one.

"I generally don't recommend a CT

scan for women unless they have risk factors and they're postmenopausal," the doctor explains. "That's when women lose the protective effect of hormones like estrogen, and risk of heart disease climbs steeply."

DAY 2: STRESS ON THE TREADMILL

We return wearing gym clothes for the treadmill stress test. "How difficult do you think it's going to be?" Stacey whispers to me in the waiting room beforehand.

"You're a yoga instructor," I reassure her. "It'll be a walk in the park." Stacey gallantly goes first—and returns dripping in sweat. "That was not a walk in the park," she says, still panting.

Moments later, it's my turn. A technician lifts my shirt and begins pressing electrode leads—flat disks backed with adhesive—all over my chest. (I'm

---

Your Best Heart Attack Prevention Plan

Arthur Agatston, MD, a preventive cardiologist, stresses lifestyle changes to all his patients, beginning with exercising regularly and maintaining a healthy weight. Although he developed the South Beach Diet—a meal plan that is rich in heart-healthy foods—to help his patients slim down and control cholesterol, he's open to any weight loss plan so long as it follows these principles.

1. Load up on good carbs (whole grains and a variety of fruits and vegetables) instead of bad carbs (white bread, pretzels, cakes, and other highly processed foods that have been stripped of fiber and nutrients).

2. Eat primarily unsaturated fats, low-fat dairy, and lean sources of protein.

3. Get an even bigger heart boost by eating at least two weekly servings of fatty fish such as tuna, salmon, or mackerel.

4. Add these especially heart-healthy foods: apples, oat bran, legumes, and, in moderation, red wine, nuts, and monounsaturated fats such as olive and canola oils.

Eat Your Way to a Healthy Heart

Here are eight picks from Arthur Agatston, MD, author of The *South Beach Heart Program*.

Apples: Research suggests that eating apples or drinking apple juice may slow the oxidation of LDL ("bad") cholesterol and help prevent plaque buildup.

How: An apple is the perfect snack. Just make sure you eat the skin, too, to get plenty of antioxidants and fiber.

Fatty Fish: The omega-3s they supply have been shown to lower triglyceride levels.

How: Put cold-water fish on the menu twice a week. Best choices are white tuna, salmon, sardines, and Spanish mackerel.

Grapefruit: It's loaded with antioxidants and soluble fiber, which help reduce heart disease.

How: Have half a grapefruit with breakfast 3 or 4 days a week.

Legumes: They lower LDL.

How: Eat hummus with raw vegetables as an afternoon snack. Or work $1/2$ cup black beans, kidney beans, lentils, red beans, or soybeans into your menu daily.

Nuts and seeds: Almonds, flaxseed, pistachios, pumpkin seeds, sesame seeds,

---

allowed to keep my bra and shirt on throughout the test.)

Then the treadmill is switched on and my heartbeat appears as a peak-shaped tracing—or electrocardiogram (EKG)—on an adjacent computer screen. As I begin striding—and while I still have my breath—I ask Dr. Agatston what this test will tell him about my cardiovascular risk.

"The heart requires anywhere from two to five times more bloodflow when you're exercising than when you're at rest," he says. "So when you're exerting yourself, we're more likely to detect compromised bloodflow, and sunflower seeds are particularly high in plant sterols, which can help reduce LDL cholesterol. Walnuts can lower triglycerides.

How: Grab 1 ounce of nuts (about a handful) for a simple midmorning or midafternoon snack. Or sprinkle some almonds or sliced walnuts on top of fat-free yogurt for dessert.

Oat bran: The soluble fiber in oat bran binds with acids in your small intestine to block the reabsorption of cholesterol.

How: For breakfast, mix 1/2 cup old-fashioned oats with 1 cup fat-free milk.

Red wine: Its phytochemicals can raise HDL ("good") cholesterol, and its polyphenols, or antioxidants, protect the lining of the coronary arteries from free-radical damage.

How: Drink a glass or two a day—but not more. Grapes are also a good source of polyphenols.

Tea: All varieties of antioxidant-rich tea can help lower LDL. Oolong tea, the kind typically served in Chinese restaurants, has been found to increase LDL particle size. That's beneficial because larger particles are less likely to enter blood vessel walls and form plaque.

How: Aim for 2 cups a day. No need to take up residence at your favorite Chinese place—oolong is available in most grocery stores.

which shows up as changes in the EKG reading."

Every few minutes, the speed of the treadmill is increased and the ramp elevated. Soon I'm too breathless to talk. Because I do 40-minute stints on an elliptical trainer a few times a week, I have little trouble completing the 20-minute test. But like Stacey, I'm glad when it's over.

DAY 3: A PEEK INSIDE OUR ARTERIES

Using an ultrasound scanner, Dr. Agatston plans to check our carotid arteries, located on either side of the neck. Unlike the coronary arteries, which are buried deep beneath the chest wall, the carotids are close to the surface, making them easy to visualize with ultrasound.

This time I go first. At the start of the test, a technician squirts gel on my neck. He then moves a device called a transducer up and down along my carotid artery—first on the left side of my neck, then on the right. I'm riveted by the ultrasound images displayed next to me on a screen. Thanks to computer enhancement, I can see blood coursing through the artery and blood moving away from the brain through an adjacent vein.

Then the technician turns on a switch, and I can hear a sound indicating blood swooshing through the artery. "That's a nice low pitch," he says. "If there's any blockage, the sound is more high-pitched."

THE TALE OF THE TAPE

At last it's time to sit down with Dr. Agatston to go over our exam results. He begins by reviewing our medical histories. The biggest risk factor for a heart attack, he tells us, is having already had a heart attack. Fortunately, neither of us fits that profile. Equally fortunate, nei-

ther of us has ever experienced the telltale symptoms of advanced coronary disease: a general weakness; faintness or breathlessness during physical exertion; or pain or a squeezing sensation in the chest, upper abdomen, or back that lasts for more than a few minutes at a time.

Next on his list of concerns is a family history of the disease. He focuses on the death of Stacey's father from heart disease at age 49.

"Early onset heart disease in your family is one of the single biggest risk factors," he says. "That's especially true if heart disease killed your father or a brother before age 55, or your mother or a sister before age 65. It's a big red flag."

"But my father was sedentary, overweight, and a heavy smoker," protests Stacey. "I'm much healthier." Without a doubt, Dr. Agatston agrees, but adds that genetics is tough to overcome. He checks our blood pressure numbers. Stacey's are an enviable 97/59. My reading is a tad higher, 112/66, but still way below what is defined as high blood pressure—a systolic (upper) number of 140 or greater and a diastolic (lower) number of 90 or more. "No problem there," Dr. Agatston says.

Both of our EKGs look perfectly normal. Dr. Agatston points to a dip—or

Move Your Body to Keep the Beat

What kind of exercise is best for your heart?

Anything that gets its rate up and keeps it there for at least 20 to 30 minutes, says Leslie Cho, MD, of the Cleveland Clinic. That generally means any aerobic activity, whether it's running, cycling, swimming, or brisk walking. The best exercises for the heart are those that "sustain your heart rate for a long time," Dr. Cho says.

Consider doing aerobic workouts several days a week and combining them with strength-training and yoga or Pilates. Your cardiovascular system will reap the rewards, and so will the rest of your body.

What's the right intensity?

When it comes to your heart, working out harder isn't necessarily better. You should aim for moderate intensity—50 to 70 percent of your maximum heart rate. A more vigorous pace won't do any damage, but you won't be able to keep it up for a long period of time. And sustaining the elevated rate is what benefits you. "You're better off doing 30 minutes of moderate exercise than 10 minutes of hard exercise," Dr. Cho says.

How do I know when I'm working out at the right intensity?

Two options. The easy way: Think of a scale from 1 to 10, with 1 being the slowest possible exercise pace and 10 the most vigorous. Aim for an intensity of 6 or 7, so you're working hard but not exhausting yourself. Or crunch some numbers: To find your target heart rate, subtract your age from 220 and multiply the result by 0.6 (for moderately intense activity). That's what you should shoot for.

Can exercising too hard cause a heart attack?

If you're already fit, no. But if you've been sedentary, doing too much too fast can put undue strain on your heart, the same way it can any muscle. "That's why we see a lot of heart attacks after the first snowstorm of the winter. People who aren't in shape go out and start shoveling," Dr. Cho says.

If you haven't been exercising at all, clear it with your doctor first. Then gradually increase how much you do.

valley—in the tracings of our heartbeats. "Sometimes we see a deeper drop, or trough, there. It's called the ST depression and can signal a blockage," he says.

Stacey and I also passed the ultrasound of our carotid arteries with flying colors. Neither of us has any visible plaque, and the inner lining of our arteries is smooth and shows no signs of thickening—indications that we have healthy vessels and are at low risk of heart attack or stroke. Stacey beams with happiness. "I guess all that yoga has paid off," she says.

Finally, he looks at the results of our blood tests. Dr. Agatston had ordered the standard blood panel we'd get with any doctor: screens for LDL ("bad" cholesterol), HDL ("good" cholesterol), triglycerides, and blood glucose levels, a test for diabetes (the disease drives up heart risk).

But that's where the similarities end. Dr. Agatston had also requested advanced blood testing for three other factors: homocysteine, an amino acid that at high levels raises your heart disease risk as much as smoking and interacts with other risk factors to hike your odds skyward; lipoprotein(a), or Lp(a), a particularly dangerous type of LDL that Dr. Agatston refers to as the widow maker because of its propensity for clogging arteries; and C-reactive protein (CRP), a marker of inflammation—in large amounts it's thought to promote the rupture of plaque. A large 2002 study in the *New England Journal of Medicine* found CRP to be a stronger predictor of heart problems in women than the standard marker, LDL cholesterol.

Dr. Agatston is happy to see that all our numbers look good. Both of us have high levels of HDL—in excess of 74 mg/dL (milligrams per deciliter of blood). "That's particularly protective," he says. A recent study shows that raising HDL by just 5 mg/dL cuts cardiovascular risk by 10 percent. "You get a lot of bang for your buck as your HDL level climbs," says Dr. Agatston.

"What about lipoprotein(a)?" I ask. "How did we do on that measure?" In his book, he describes this particle as a major villain that could sometimes "explain plaque buildup seen in heart scans of patients who have seemingly normal cholesterol levels." Humoring me, he double-checks the numbers and reassures us our levels are low.

Stacey and I are beginning to look like twins—very healthy twins. Despite similar results, however, Dr. Agatston ranks my risk at less than 10 percent (meaning 90 percent of people my age are more likely to get heart disease) and Stacey's at 20 percent—low but double mine.

"It's because she has a family history of the disease and you don't," he says. For that reason, he recommends that Stacey come back for further testing after she hits menopause. As for me, he says: "Unless you develop high blood pressure or other risk factors, I won't need to see you again."

Good news all around, but what if we hadn't aced all those tests? I want to know. Then what?

The first challenge for patients is to improve their diet and begin exercising, says Dr. Agatston. (See "Six Steps to a Healthy Heart," page 247, for more information.) But, he warns, "you can only get so far with diet and exercise—genes count, too." That's why he argues that anyone with risk factors should have all the tests he performed on Stacey and me done by age 50—or even earlier if there's familial heart disease at a young age.

"If the results from those exams raise any further concerns, I may also order a heart scan," he says. "Then I sit down with the patient and recommend a series of interventions tailored to his or her specific needs."

For patients with high LDL or CRP scores, statin drugs can work well, he reports. "They're usually very well tolerated and can virtually stop atherosclerosis in its tracks," he tells us. "I just saw a 65-year-old woman whose cholesterol levels and other risk factors have been tightly controlled over the past 10 years. A recent heart scan shows no new plaque above the level recorded at the time of her first scan 7 years ago."

Other powerful interventions include prescription-strength niacin pills, for raising low HDL levels; aspirin, for countering inflammation and thinning the blood; a prescription fish-oil supplement, for improving the overall health of the vessels and stabilizing irregular heartbeats; and a variety of medications for controlling high blood pressure and diabetes.

THE SKEPTICS' VIEW

By the end of our consultation with Dr. Agatston, Stacey and I can't help being swayed by his perspective. But not all cardiologists agree that the research is far enough along to justify the extra expense of all the testing he proposes.

"There's no question the health system is reactive rather than proactive toward heart disease when it comes to identifying and treating people at moderate risk," says cardiologist Clyde W. Yancy, MD, medical director of Baylor Heart and Vascular Institute in Dallas and a spokesperson for the American Heart Association. He respects what Dr. Agatston is doing but thinks it's too soon to be making blanket recommendations about screening tests. In his opinion, that kind of judgment call has to be made case by case, based on individual risk factors.

Dr. Yancy also cautions that preventive health care is still in its infancy. "We need to fund much more research aimed at clarifying our understanding and treatment of the new risk factors—things like homocysteine and C-reactive protein," he says.

At the Women's Heart Clinic at the Mayo Clinic in Rochester, Minnesota, director Sharonne Hayes, MD, agrees with Dr. Yancy. "Testing for Lp(a), homocysteine, and CRP has not yet been shown to improve a patient's chances of living longer," she says. "They can help us understand what sort of risks someone is facing. I use the same tests in my practice every day. But until we have definitive proof, I think we have to be much more selective about who gets these tests. If we screened everybody, we'd break the bank."

Dr. Hayes isn't kidding: The total bill for all six tests Dr. Agatston recommends runs about $2,000. Right now, insurance would cover only a small portion of that bill, though Dr. Agatston expects that to change as more research findings prove the tests' value.

Nonetheless, Jay N. Cohn, MD, director of the Rasmussen Center for Cardiovascular Disease Prevention at the University of Minnesota, is more aligned with Dr. Agatston's stance. Although he acknowledges the controversy about the best screening methods, he believes "there's agreement that we need to be doing a much better job at identifying people in need of early intervention." Echoing Dr. Agatston's words, he adds, "With good preventive care, heart attacks can be virtually eliminated."

Dr. Agatston has heard his peers' concerns—and he agrees. Many of the screens are for those with already established risks of heart disease. That's why Stacey and I didn't get the CT scan, no matter how much we may have wanted it. He also agrees that research should continue on things like homocysteine and Lp(a), so that doctors can further refine diagnosis and treatment. But he feels strongly that it's time we start spending our health care dollars more wisely.

"As a society, we're investing the bulk of our money in bypass surgery, angioplasty, and other expensive, aggressive late-stage treatments for heart disease," he says. Wouldn't it be better to spend that money on making sure people never have a heart attack in the first place?

"The tests aren't cheap," he concedes, "but if you think of them as an investment in our future, they're a bargain."

Six Steps to a Healthy Heart

"It's important to take care of your heart even before you have any symptoms," says Arthur Agatston, MD, a preventive cardiologist. "Quite simply, the earlier you start, the easier it is to prevent heart disease."

Luckily, the latest research shows that the road to a healthy heart isn't so rough. Here, six steps to make sure your beat goes on for a long, long time.

Step 1: So, How's Your Mom?

Researchers have long believed that having a close family member (mom, dad, sister, or brother) with cardiovascular disease is one of the clearest predictors of heart trouble in your own future. But according to a 2006 Swedish study, it's really Mom you need to worry about. Your risk increases by 17 percent if your father has heart disease, but it shoots up by a whopping 43 percent if your mother is afflicted.

This may be more environment than genetics, since children typically spend more time with their mothers and tend to learn lifestyle habits from them. But even if you don't smoke and you do exercise, it's possible that your risk could still be up as much as 82 percent if both of your parents had heart disease.

Which doesn't mean you're doomed, of course. But it does mean you shouldn't

(continued)

Six Steps to a Healthy Heart (cont.)

waste any time. If you have a family history, Dr. Agatston recommends in-depth tests that go beyond the normal blood workup every few years, starting in your midforties. First, talk to your doctor about having a CT scan of your heart, which can detect attack-causing plaque buildup in your arteries—even years in advance. The first one establishes a baseline; subsequent images assess potential deterioration of the arteries.

Although the scans aren't typically covered by insurance, that may change in the next few years. In the meantime, many hospitals and clinics accept payment plans. "The extra expense is worth it to prevent heart disease," Dr. Agatston says. "These are tests that really can make a difference in people's lives."

Dr. Agatston also suggests that all women request more detailed blood tests that measure not only the level of cholesterol but its type and size—factors that he says affect the heart in ways that scientists are only now beginning to understand. Talk to your doctor about a standard lipid profile. A blood test can also detect the presence of C-reactive protein in the bloodstream, which may contribute to plaque formation. More prevalent in people who are overweight, sedentary, hypertensive, or smokers, C-reactive protein's presence accurately predicts the likelihood of heart attacks in women with relatively low cholesterol, and researchers speculate that it could signal heart disease before symptoms develop. Ask your doctor to check your numbers next time you get blood work done.

Step 2: Sorry, You're Gonna Have to Do a Little Math

The connection between cholesterol—a waxy substance made in your liver and found in blood cells—and heart disease has been known for decades, but your total cholesterol number is only part of the equation. The real key is how much of it is low-density lipoprotein (LDL), the so-called bad cholesterol, and how much is high-density lipoprotein (HDL), the "good" kind.

LDL cholesterol can build up in your arterial walls, causing plaque, which can rupture in the arteries and result in blood clots and possibly heart attacks. A recent study from the University of Texas Southwestern Medical Center indicates that keeping LDL levels low (the longer the better) can protect even people with other risk factors like smoking. Meanwhile, HDL plays the role of crime-fighting superhero to LDL's nasty villain, transporting the bad stuff through the blood to the liver, where it's metabolized and then eliminated. A Mayo Clinic newsletter article indicated that increasing HDL by even 1 milligram per deciliter (mg/dL) can reduce heart attack risk by 3 percent. "Basically, you want more of the good stuff, less of the bad stuff," says Sharonne Hayes, MD, director of the Mayo Clinic Women's Heart Clinic.

For most people, total cholesterol should be under 200, with LDL levels no higher than 100 and HDL no lower than 40 for men and 50 for women. If your numbers are in line, doctors recommend retesting your blood every 5 years in your twenties and thirties.

Step 3: Don't Be Afraid to Do Drugs

If blood tests show your cholesterol is high, a change in diet and exercise might help (see steps 5 and 6 for some suggestions). But in many cases, it's too late or your numbers are too high for these basic steps to help.

That's when your doctor may give you a cholesterol-lowering medication, known as a statin, which keeps the liver from producing too much cholesterol. Some doctors have questioned the wisdom of prescribing these drugs, especially for patients who might lower their cholesterol through lifestyle changes. But recent studies show that statins can diminish LDL by as much as 40 percent, slightly raise the level of HDL, and reduce the risk of heart attacks by about 35 percent. This is why many experts say these medications are actually underprescribed.

"Statins are incredible tools in lowering cholesterol and can keep many people

(continued)

Six Steps to a Healthy Heart (cont.)

from suffering heart attacks," Dr. Agatston says. "But there's no question: They're meant to work together with proper diet and exercise."

People taking statins may experience muscle fatigue as a side effect, though, and should get regular blood tests to check liver function.

Step 4: Ask Yourself, "What Kind of Fruit Am I?"

Carrying extra weight around isn't just a drag during swimsuit season. It can also be dangerous, especially if those excess pounds find their way to your belly and not, say, your hips. Recent studies indicate that abdominal fat is metabolically different from the other fat in your body: As you gain padding around your middle, the individual cells swell, and their size is linked to higher triglyceride levels and lower good cholesterol.

The best treatment for belly fat? Signing up for Weight Watchers isn't enough; you're going to have to pry yourself off the couch, too. New research from Wake Forest University Baptist Medical Center shows that diet and exercise together reduce the size of abdominal fat cells, which doesn't happen if you lose weight through dieting alone. Working out regularly also has a ripple effect on the body: Not only do dangerous pounds come off, but your muscles become more efficient at using blood; your heart gets stronger; and your blood vessels become more limber, so blood flows more easily.

"A lot of things don't make you feel better in the short term," Dr. Hayes says. "Exercise is the one thing that does."

And you don't have to run a marathon every week to get these benefits. Cardiologists recommend an average of 30 minutes of moderate aerobic exercise a day, which has been shown to increase life expectancy by $3^1/_2$ years. Whether walking, running, or swimming, you should aim to work your heart to about 50 to 70 percent of its maximum rate. Even this amount of exercise is powerful enough to combat other high-risk factors: A study out of the Cooper Institute in Dallas found that even moderately fit people had half the death rates of those who were sedentary.

While doctors used to think that weight-training was bad for the heart because it increased blood pressure, research now shows it can actually lower blood pressure when transforming fat into muscle, which burns calories and keeps them from landing on your belly. This is why Nieca Goldberg, MD, a New York City cardiologist and author of *The Women's Healthy Heart Program*, recommends strengthening exercises two or three times a week for all the major muscle groups—arms, legs, shoulders, chest, back, hips, and trunk.

Dr. Agatston suggests a Pilates- or yoga-based regimen that zeroes in on the core muscles of your abdomen and lower back. Either way, consistency is key, as is starting young: Dr. Goldberg says regular strengthening can not only help prevent age-related loss of bone and muscle mass but also help reduce body fat and improve endurance, both of which can decrease your risk of heart disease.

Step 5: Hey, Are Those Your Arteries Closing Up?

Exercise without diet gets you only halfway to where you need to be. But changing the way you eat doesn't mean starving yourself or signing up for a fad diet.

"There's no single food that's going to kill you or save your life," Dr. Hayes says. "Proper diet is about a wide variety of healthy foods." That means, most important, avoiding trans and saturated fats: In a 2006 Australian study, researchers found that giving healthy subjects just one fatty meal affected bloodflow and diminished HDL's protective qualities.

In its latest dietary recommendations, the American Heart Association suggests that no more than 7 percent of your daily calories come from saturated fats—butter, full-fat dairy such as whole milk or cheese, and meat. Meanwhile, only 1 percent of your daily diet should consist of trans fats, which are found mostly in processed foods such as cookies, crackers, and chips.

(continued)

Six Steps to a Healthy Heart (cont.)

This is why Dr. Goldberg encourages sticking to a "Mediterranean" diet: a moderate amount of foods high in unsaturated fats such as olive oil and fish; lean meat, such as beef fillet, flank, or sirloin, and pork tenderloin; low-fat dairy; whole grains (think brown rice and barley); and at least five daily servings of colorful fruits and vegetables, which provide antioxidants that help keep blood vessels flexible.

In particular, Dr. Goldberg and others tout the benefits of omega-3 fatty acids, found in salmon and other fish, because they may help lower blood pressure and the risk of abnormal heart rhythms. Dr. Agatston also recommends incorporating foods that lower bad cholesterol, like apples, which research suggests may help prevent plaque buildup; oolong tea, which has strong antioxidant properties that can make LDL particles bigger and less likely to enter the bloodstream; and legumes, such as beans, peas, and lentils, which decrease risk of cardiovascular disease. And he suggests foods such as almonds and walnuts and up to two glasses a day of red wine, which help reduce LDL cholesterol and protect the lining of the arteries.

Step 6: Stop Saying That an Occasional Cigarette Won't Hurt

Yes, you've heard the antismoking rant before. But there's a reason for it. Quitting smoking should top your list of things to do to avoid heart disease, Dr. Hayes says. And that's true even if the only time you light up is over mojitos with friends.

Recent research shows that smoking between one and five cigarettes a day triples your chance of dying from a heart attack, and that it's even worse for women than for men. Smoking narrows arteries, raises blood pressure, thickens blood, and makes it more likely to clot—the classic recipe for a heart attack. This is especially true if you have other risk factors, such as high blood pressure and high cholesterol, which together with smoking make you much more likely to get heart disease, according to Dr. Agatston. You take birth control and smoke? You've just put another bullet in the gun. That combo raises blood pressure and can lead to blood clots, further increasing your risk.

CHAPTER 26

BLUES CLUES

If you're taking an antidepressant, chances are you've gone off your meds a few times. But new research shows that's no way to beat the blues. Here's a smarter Rx for feeling like yourself again

According to the American Diabetes Association, people with diabetes have a greater risk of depression than people without diabetes. On the flip side, people who are depressed are more likely to get type 2 diabetes.

The National Center for Health Statistics notes that antidepressants are the most prescribed class of drugs following doctors visits. But here's the irony: Statistics show that a whopping 60 percent of people who begin popping one of these pills on Memorial Day will have given up by Labor Day. Some quit because of side effects such as a throbbing head, tighter jeans, or a sucker-punched libido. (It's a cruel irony that these minuses often start in just days, while the feel-good benefits can take weeks to kick in.) Others stop when their depression lets up, figuring they've got it beat.

Drug Buy

According to a 6-year study, only 30 percent of patients recovered from depression with the first antidepressant they tried. (Two-thirds recovered after a second, third, or fourth attempt.) But even if you find a good fix, stats show that you won't stick with it if the side effects suck.

Here are eight meds that succeeded in reducing at least half of depression symptoms in most people who took them—plus what percentage of patients ended up quitting the drugs. Costs are for the average month, before insurance. For the full report, go to www.crbestbuydrugs.org.

DRUG NAME	BUPROPION (WELLBUTRIN)	CITALOPRAM (CELEXA)	ESCITALOPRAM (LEXAPRO)	DULOXETINE (CYMBALTA)
Quit Rate	6–8 percent	5–9 percent	3–10 percent	3–13 percent
Cost	$62–90	$44–46	$96–100	$131–293

DRUG NAME	FLUOXETINE (PROZAC, SARAFEM)	SERTRALINE (ZOLOFT)	PAROXETINE (PAXIL)	VENLAFAXINE (EFFEXOR)
Quit Rate	7–14 percent	7–14 percent	7–16 percent	9–16 percent
Cost	$33–66	$85	$64	$132

Note: Quit rates reflect the range found in studies of each drug.

The thing is, lots of people will wind up grabbing the pill bottle again—maybe more than once. Though there are no hard stats, anecdotal evidence suggests that women are increasingly treating antidepressants like Advil: We go on them when we feel bad, stop when we feel better (or when the side effects bum us out), and go on them again if the blues come back.

But new research shows that an on-again, off-again relationship with antidepressants can have far more repercussions than anyone realized.

A DRUG HOLIDAY

Now that antidepressants are as commonly dispensed as PEZ, it's easy to forget that most are less than 20 years old. Prozac, the first SSRI (selective serotonin reuptake inhibitor; these keep the happy chemical serotonin in your brain longer) was launched in 1987, the same year Patrick Swayze swiveled his hips in *Dirty Dancing*. Now antidepressants are a $12.6 billion business, and, according to health care company Medco Health Solutions, 90 percent of the prescriptions are for SSRIs, including Lexapro, Paxil, and Zoloft, or for their close cousins, SNRIs (serotonin and norepinephrine reuptake inhibitors) such as Cymbalta and Effexor.

If you're on an SSRI, you've probably skipped a random Saturday or tried life sans Lexapro for a week, just to see if you could thrive without the drug. "Everybody does it either a little or a lot," says psychiatrist Eve Wood, MD, author of 10 *Steps to Take Charge of Your Emo-*

tional Life, "because everybody would rather not be on medication, and, understandably, no one likes the idea of being on drugs for the rest of their life."

One of the urban myths that persist among patients (and a few doctors) is that it's fine to take a little drug holiday, especially if the meds are making you as interested in sex as a spayed collie. Here's how it works, in theory at least: You take your last dose of the week on Thursday morning and don't start again until Sunday at noon. In between, you enjoy hours of lovemaking that would put the horniest starlet to shame. Most doctors, however, don't agree that this is an Rx for ecstasy. "The libido is very complicated," says David Baron, DO, chair of the department of psychiatry at Temple University School of Medicine. He doubts it's capable of bouncing back after a mere 24- or 48-hour drug boycott. What may bounce back, however, is your depression.

The truth is, taking a break could work for some people. Or it might not. Experts still don't know exactly how antidepressants work, in part because we don't really understand depression. What's clear so far is this: Major depression is elusive and ever changing, a perfect storm of family history, environment, life events, and all the idiosyncrasies of your wiring. It doesn't even make sense to talk about depression as a single disorder, says Gerald Sanacora, MD, PhD, director of the Yale University School of Medicine Depression Research Program: "It's more of a syndrome, with multiple causes and paths of physiology." So if you've got a severe case, skipping a few days of your meds can bring the black cloud back. That's especially true if you're on a drug that flushes out of your system quickly, such as Paxil or Zoloft. Prozac, on the other hand, lingers in the bloodstream for a couple of weeks, which makes a Prozac holiday pointless.

I CAN'T QUIT YOU

No one can predict what life will look and feel like once you stop the pills. Take Caleigh Wright (not her real name), 27, a university administrator in the South who began taking Prozac in college when she found herself sleeping 16 hours a day to escape anxiety. A few years ago, she decided to experience life unmedicated. "I wanted to be able to say, 'Hey, I'm a strong woman, I don't need drugs,'" she recalls. When she quit Pro-

zac, though, her symptoms returned in a couple of weeks. "I felt desperately down in the dumps," she says, "and I'd get these intense anxiety spikes over the smallest things," like a party where she didn't know everyone, even a conversation with friends about her career. She returned to the drug within weeks, then repeated this scenario a few more times, hoping each time her depression would be gone. "I've finally just come to accept that I have these wonky brain molecules that need help marinating in serotonin," she says.

Wright was lucky: For her, Prozac still packed its same punch. Because when you toss your pills, says Madhukar Trivedi, MD, a leading depression researcher at the Mood Disorders Research Program and Clinic at the University of Texas Southwestern Medical Center, "you run the risk that if your depression comes back, the same treatment won't work." No one really knows why the pill that worked once might not the second (or third) time around. But it's not that you've developed a tolerance to the drug, Dr. Wood says. Instead, your brain chemistry could have changed. "Depression has a life of its own," she explains. "It can shift enough that an intervention that once worked no longer does. And that's when you need to tweak the dose or consider a different medication."

Dr. Baron hypothesizes that when a pill poops out, it's because your system is now more vulnerable to depression, especially if you weren't on a high enough dose to begin with or didn't take it long enough. It's like a sprained ankle, he says: "If you go back in the game after icing the injury only a half hour, the ankle hasn't had a chance to heal. It also takes less stress for you to sprain the ankle again." So when treatment isn't adequate and consistent, you can get depressed again more easily, and it can take you longer to recover. In fact, cycling on and off can actually make your depression resistant to treatment.

STOP SIGNS

Okay, but it also doesn't make any sense to take a drug you no longer need. And the good news is that lots of people do stop needing antidepressants. If you've had one episode of clinical depression, there's a fifty-fifty chance you'll never have another. If your depression comes back, though, there's a 70 percent chance it will come back a third time, too. Once you've had three episodes,

the odds that you'll have another soar to 90 percent.

So the latest medical guidelines go like this: The first time you're diagnosed with clinical depression, stay on antidepressants for 6 to 9 months. (The average depressive episode lasts about 9 months.) When you begin to wonder if it's time to be drug free, ask yourself: "Have my moods—and life—been stable for a few months? Have I made concrete, positive changes, such as finding a saner job or taking up a walking program?" When you can answer yes to both, talk to your MD about quitting.

Once you have the green light, you'll taper off your meds for a couple of weeks to several months. Unlike the cold-turkey approach, gradually weaning off the drugs helps you avoid withdrawal symptoms such as dizziness, nausea, anxiety, and headaches, and it diminishes the potential for rebound effects.

Next, create a checklist of very specific depressive symptoms that you've suffered in the past—say, crashing for 10 or 12 hours every night; losing interest in tennis, sex, and molten chocolate cake; starting heated arguments about who caused the paper jam in the office copier; sobbing during commercial breaks of

Men in Trees. Be prepared to discuss a return to antidepressants if these symptoms linger for more than a few days. Finally, enlist a close friend as your emotional watchdog.

"You might think you're just having a bad few days or that work isn't going well," says Nada Stotland, MD, a Chicago-based psychiatrist, "but this person who knows you well will be able to say, 'It's coming back.'"

Once your doc finds a drug (or drugs) that works for you this time (see "Drug Buy" on page 254), stay on it for 1 to 2 years to provide a few extra months of insurance against relapse. "It's not like treating an infection with an antibiotic," Dr. Baron says. And if you feel depressed again after that? "You're looking at long-term or possibly lifetime treatment."

WALK THE TALK

Whether this is your first or third time battling depression, you don't need to rely on pharmaceuticals alone. New research shows that combining antidepressants with cognitive behavioral therapy (CBT) can have a near-kryptonite effect on the black dog. CBT is a short-term (just 16 to 20 sessions), no-nonsense approach to therapy with a straightforward goal: to help people unlearn depressive ways of thinking. For example, depressed women tend to catastrophize ("Oh my God, my boss said I need to punch up my presentation—I'm going to lose my job!") and to attribute setbacks to unfixable flaws ("I always become a stammering, sweaty mess when I speak to more than three coworkers at once"). With cognitive therapy, patients learn that they've been clinging to a hugely distorted, very unflattering story about themselves that doesn't reflect reality, says Zindel Segal, PhD, a leading CBT researcher in Toronto.

A recent 3-year study found that among 700 people who were chronically depressed, 85 percent improved significantly—or saw their depression disappear altogether—after just 12 weeks of an SSRI plus CBT. Brain scans show that drugs work on the subcortical regions, where emotions are processed, while therapy changes the prefrontal cortex, where the brain processes information. Which means you're taking two routes to recovery at the same time. We feel better already.

CHAPTER 27

THE CANCER CONNECTION

A growing stack of research confirms a chilling link: People with type 2 diabetes are at slightly higher risk of a variety of cancers. Here's how to protect yourself

"Diabetics' high insulin levels can spur the growth of cancer cells and even cause normal cells to dangerously mutate and multiply," says Tim Byers, MD, deputy director of the University of Colorado Cancer Center, who presented his findings at a recent American Diabetes Association conference.

The effect isn't limited to people with diabetes, he says. Anything that raises insulin production—especially being overweight or inactive—can increase cancer risk, too. Research shows a link between diabetes and several types of cancer, including breast, uterine, colon, pancreatic, and liver.

The good news: People with diabetes who keep their blood sugar low with diet and exercise can sidestep the added cancer danger. And, of course, they can follow the same advice as people without diabetes to reduce their overall cancer risk.

NO-HYPE CANCER FIGHTERS

So you gave up charred meats, you're using your gym membership, and you ingest enough fiber to choke Wilford Brimley. Because you know what's good for you. But every time you turn on the news, you're hit with more advice on how to prevent cancer. Some of it is common sense (don't smoke), while some sounds as dubious as Britney Spears's parenting techniques (eat ground red pepper). With all the studies and hype, we wouldn't blame you for feeling confused.

The good news: You can prevent 50 to 70 percent of cancers by exercising more, chucking cigarettes, and improving your diet, says Therese Bevers, MD, medical director for M. D. Anderson's Cancer Prevention Center in Houston. Plus, you have a better chance if you start now. That's because cell mutations—which are how cancer gets going—can begin decades before a tumor appears, says Cynthia Stein, MD, coauthor of *Handbook of Cancer Risk Assessment and Prevention*. To find the most tried-and-true ways to a cancer-free future, we plowed through piles of research and talked to leading cancer experts. Here are the lucky four.

TAKE A HISTORY LESSON

You know your Scottish grandfather's tartan pattern and your grandmother's maiden name, but how well do you know their health histories? Just 5 to 10 percent of cancer cases are related to your genetic inheritance, but if you do carry an unlucky gene, your risk of getting that cancer is enormous (50 to 100 percent), Dr. Bevers says. Three of the most common types—breast, ovarian, and colorectal—seem to have the strongest genetic link.

Prevention prescription: Take down your family's medical history, noting the disease and when each relative was diagnosed. (The earlier the age of a cancer diagnosis and the more relatives who've had it, the stronger your family history.) Be sure to get info on both sides: You have the same chance of inheriting the genes from Mom and from Dad, even for breast and ovarian cancers, Dr. Bevers says.

If your family tree shows a history of cancer, consider talking to a genetic counselor, who may recommend tests, suggests Ted Gansler, MD, director of medical content for the American Cancer Society (ACS). But keep in mind that even if a test says you have the gene, no one can predict for certain whether you'll get cancer, he cautions.

Knowing you're at increased risk may mean you get screenings like mammograms or colonoscopies sooner or more often than someone without a strong family history, says Axel Goetz, MD, PhD, chief science officer at RealAge.com, a consumer health media company. And let's face it: You've got a no-brainer incentive to make anticancer lifestyle changes a priority if you know your genetic risk is high.

KNOW YOUR BOOZE CLUES

Though studies touting red wine's benefits—a stronger ticker, better memory, longer life, and even possibly cancer prevention—come out about as often as Brad Pitt adopts a kid, that doesn't mean an open bar is a prescription for health. While a single glass of vino is probably good (thanks mostly to resveratrol, an antioxidant in grapes that protects cells against free radicals, the unstable molecules that damage them), studies indicate that women who throw back two or more cocktails a day up their breast cancer risk by about 40 percent.

Why? "Alcohol increases the liver's production of estrogen, and the more estrogen in your body, the greater your risk of getting cancer," says Wendy Chen, MD, an oncologist and epidemiologist at Harvard Medical School.

Prevention prescription: You can undo some of the consequences of girls' night out by popping a multivitamin with 400 micrograms of folic acid. When you drink, your body turns alcohol into a carcinogen that hurts the DNA in cells, but folic acid seems to help repair the damage. Researchers say 400 micrograms will counterbalance the effects of only one drink, though. The bottom line? "With one drink per day, the benefits of red wine are in balance with the harms, so it's okay to have a glass with dinner," Dr. Goetz says.

SWEAT MORE—AND MORE OFTEN

Exercise doesn't just tone your muscles and help you shrug off the stress of your boss's daily diatribe. The latest research shows that working out does a lot more to protect you from cancer than doctors previously thought.

"Exercise reduces the amount of hormones in your body like insulin growth factors, which make small tumors grow faster and get bigger than they would otherwise," says Gary Bennett, PhD, assistant professor at the Dana-Farber Cancer Institute in Boston.

Regular sweat sessions also strengthen your immune system so it's better equipped to destroy germs and cancerous cells, adds Colleen Doyle, RD, director of nutrition and physical activity at the ACS. Trouble is, most of us aren't getting anywhere near the society's recommended 30 minutes of moderate to vigorous exercise at least 5 days a week.

Prevention prescription: Start by fessing up to how much and how intensely you're really exercising. Many people overestimate their daily physical activity (shoe shopping or a sprint to the weekly staff meeting doesn't count), Dr. Bennett says. To reap the greatest cancer-fighting rewards, 45 to 60 minutes of heart-pumping activity most days of the week is your best bet.

PUT PLANTS ON YOUR PLATE

Scientists have yet to determine the benefits of a diet rich in peanut butter M&M'S, but they continue to find more reasons to load up on produce. It's safe to say that you know that fruits and veggies are supercharged with antioxidants and phytochemicals that mop up free radicals. A study from Children's Hospital Oakland Research Institute in California found that without enough of these good guys, cells find it so hard to Swiffer themselves that their defenses weaken, making you more vulnerable to cancer.

Prevention prescription: There's no cancer-preventing RDA for antioxidants and phytochemicals (a cup of berries has hundreds), but eating five to nine servings of produce a day seems to be your best defense. (What's a serving? A piece of fruit, half a cup of cooked or raw veggies, or a cup of raw leafy greens.) Eat a wide variety of produce, recommends Dr. Goetz, and get the most bang for the bunch by shopping with an eye for color—from deep greens (such as spinach and kale) and purples and blues (eggplant, berries) to oranges (carrots, sweet potatoes) and reds (bell peppers, strawberries). "The more colorful ingredients you eat," he says, "the greater the preventive effect."

The Next Big Things?

Soy, beta-carotene, vitamin E—they're the disappointments of the cancer-fighting world. They had such potential but so far have failed to deliver, sometimes even doing more harm than good. But for every disappointment, there's a success story. Here are two promising cancer weapons to watch.

Vitamin D

Call it a triple threat: Vitamin D encourages abnormal cells to die, improves immunity, and stops the blood vessels needed to grow a tumor, says researcher William Grant, PhD. One study found that people who got at least 600 IU (400 is the Daily Value) every day had a 41 percent lower risk of pancreatic cancer than those who got less than 150 IU. Don't rely on the most direct source of D—the sun's rays—because that raises your skin cancer risk. Instead, get 400 to 1,000 IU from a daily supplement or foods such as milk, egg yolks, salmon, tuna, and D-fortified cereal.

Sleep

You probably go from Conan to Soledad without a solid 8 hours of shut-eye. Research shows that exposure to light at night ups your cancer risk: One Harvard study found night-shift workers had a 23 percent greater risk of breast cancer. It may be because your brain releases the hormone melatonin, which inhibits cancer cells, only in darkness, says Tulane University's Steven Hill, PhD. Get your 8 hours nightly, in complete darkness. That means no lights (including a TV or computer) during wee-hours bathroom trips; just seconds of exposure to light can stop melatonin production.

MEDICAL BREAKTHROUGHS

Diabetes can usher many unwelcome complications into your life besides heart disease, depression, and cancer. For example, researchers from the American Association of Clinical Endocrinologists say type 2 diabetes can boost your risk of kidney disease by 22 percent, eye damage by 19 percent, foot problems by 13 percent, heart attack by 8 percent, congestive heart failure by 7 percent, and stroke by 5 percent. Here's the latest research on some of these unwelcome diabetes complications.

THE DIABETES-PARKINSON'S CONNECTION

Finnish researchers have turned up a disturbing link between diabetes and Parkinson's disease, the nervous system disorder that leads to muscle tremors and paralysis. In an 18-year study that tracked 51,552 healthy individuals with no family history of the disease, those who developed diabetes were twice as likely to end up with Parkinson's as those without diabetes.

No one's sure what the connection is yet, but it's possible that receptors for the neurotransmitter dopamine—which helps direct muscles—may be impaired in diabetics, says study author Jaakko Tuomilehto, MD, a professor at the University of Helsinki. Whatever the link, he recommends that people with diabetes and their doctors be alert to the potential risk and watch for symptoms—trembling limbs, body stiffness, and loss of balance and coordination.

POP THESE PILLS FOR PAIN?

A supplement called acetyl L-carnitine (ALC) claims to relieve diabetic neuropathy: pain and numbness caused by nerve damage. (Acetyl L-carnitine is different from L-carnitine that athletes take to increase endurance.)

But does it work? That's a definite maybe. Some studies show pain relief and possible nerve regeneration. The good news is that side effects are rare and mild, primarily nausea. The bad news is that ALC can interfere with multiple medications. The dosage is 500 milligrams, three times a day, but take it only under a doctor's supervision.

ENJOY THE WEEKEND

Protect your heart the fun way: Savor your Saturdays and Sundays. Finnish researchers asked 788 workers about their ability to relax on the weekends and then tracked them for 28 years. Those who said they seldom or rarely felt renewed, alert, and ready to head back to work by Monday morning were about three times as likely to die of heart disease or stroke.

Stress can damage hormones, nerves, and the immune system; chronic stress, such as that from a job, may increase that wear and tear, says lead researcher Mika Kivimäki, PhD. If you're having trouble unwinding, make it a priority to get some time for yourself. And consider talking to your manager about shifting some of your workload or whether you can arrange an alternate schedule, like part- or flextime.

FEED YOUR HEART

Start eating magnesium-rich foods early in life and your heart will benefit years later, new Northwestern University research shows. Magnesium is in lots of luscious foods, including these.

MAGNESIUM SOURCES	MILLIGRAMS PER SERVING
Pumpkin seeds, 1 oz	151
Halibut, 3 oz	91
Spinach, cooked, 1/2 c	78
Almonds, 1 oz	78
Cashews, 1 oz	77
Pine nuts, 1 oz	71
Tuna, 3 oz	54
Peanuts, 1 oz	50
Artichokes, 1/2 c	50
Soy milk, 8 oz	47
Yogurt, 8 oz	43
Brown rice, 1/2 c	42
Sunflower seeds, 1 oz	41

INSTANT DEPRESSION CURE?

Instant relief from unrelenting depression may someday be just a pinprick away. A small study conducted by the National Institutes of Health suggests that an injection of the anesthetic ketamine may help people who don't respond to antidepressant drugs.

Researchers recruited 18 men and women whose symptoms had resisted standard treatment. After a single dose of ketamine, more than half reported that their feelings improved substantially within 2 hours; 71 percent felt their moods lighten within a day. And the lift lasted—a week for about a third of participants. Traditional antidepressants, which help only about 50 percent of users, can take several weeks to be effective and must be swallowed daily.

Experts suspect that typical antidepressants target brain circuits that only indirectly affect depression. Ketamine seems to get closer to the source, says lead author Carlos A. Zarate Jr., MD. Next up: a longer-term study of its safety and effectiveness.

DEPRESSION MYTHS, BUSTED

Roughly 15 million Americans suffer from depression, and many let misperceptions hinder their recovery. A new survey of 1,200 women by the National Women's Health Resource Center and drugmaker Eli Lilly exposes common myths by generation.

20- to 44-year-olds tend to say...

Myth: "I don't need antidepressants—I can lean on my friends to help get me through this."

Truth: You will need more than a pal to beat depression.

"Friends and family are key to recovery—but people with serious depression respond best if they also receive talk therapy and an antidepressant," says Vivian Burt, MD, PhD, a professor emeritus of psychiatry at the David Geffen School of Medicine at UCLA.

45- to 59-year-olds claim...

Myth: "It's not depression; it's a menopausal mood swing."

Truth: Menopause isn't a reason for not seeking treatment.

"Regardless of what sends you into depression—and menopause can—you need real remedies," Dr. Burt says.

60- to 69-year-olds often believe...

Myth: "It's best not to burden others with my problems."

Truth: Talking to friends—in addition to a therapist—will help considerably when it comes to beating the blues.

"There's a stigma with depression for this age group," Dr. Burt says. "Older women may feel ashamed and vulnerable, which is why they need social support."

BLUE GENES

Keep your head up: If someone in your immediate family suffered from chronic major depression before age 31, you have more than double the average risk of getting hit with it yourself. That's the finding of a Johns Hopkins University–led study of more than 600 people and their families. What's more, if one of your siblings, parents, or children battled the blues before age 13, your risk rises sixfold.

Study author James Potash, MD, MPH, recommends that people with this family history alert a doctor if they notice failing energy, a pattern of insomnia or oversleeping, decreased appetite, or a general sense of dissatisfaction or sadness. Also, limiting alcohol consumption and stress can help stabilize your mood.

DILIGENCE FIXES DEPRESSION

Beating depression is like buying shoes: You have to keep trying new options until you find the right fit. According to a new 3,671-person study—the nation's largest ever on depression treatments—only 37 percent reported relief with the first method, the drug citalopram, which belongs to the class of the most commonly prescribed antidepressants. It took three more tries for a total of 67 percent of the patients to recover.

"Most treatments take up to 12 weeks to fully kick in," says Madhukar Trivedi, MD, director of the mood disorders program at the University of Texas Southwestern Medical Center. Consider tracking your moods and discussing the results with your physician.

POSE THESE QUESTIONS

Women are more likely to know Mom's family history of breast cancer than Dad's, finds a recent Virginia Commonwealth University study. But both sides figure in your risk. Ask both of your parents these three questions.

1. Did a family member have cancer at a young age—especially breast cancer before 50?
2. Did any men have breast cancer?
3. Did anyone have multiple cancers? Nonbreast cancers count: Some gene mutations that raise breast risk can also cause several other cancers.

CHEAT A LITTLE

Here's a reason to grin: Even your favorite off-limit treats kick in toward your choline goal of 425 milligrams. Why care about choline? In recent USDA research, the nutrient lowered blood levels of homocysteine by 8 percent, a sign of protection from cancer, heart attack, stroke, and dementia. Pack your diet with wheat germ (43 milligrams in $1/4$ cup), baked beans (40 in $1/2$ cup), and pistachios (22 in $1/4$ cup). But these surprising choline sources can help, too.

THE CHEAT	THE CHOLINE
Chocolate cake, 1-in. slice	162 mg
Blueberry muffin	59 mg
Chicken nuggets, 6 pieces	39 mg
Beef-and-bean burrito, 3.5 oz	28 mg
Light beer, 8 oz	19 mg
Vanilla ice cream, $1/2$ c	19 mg

PART VII

DIABETES COOKBOOK

CHAPTER 28

THE RECIPES

Control your blood sugar with these 100 diabetes-friendly recipes

You—and your family—will love these delicious, nutritious recipes. Besides tasting good, they're good for you.

When selecting these recipes, we divided the FDA's daily value for calories—2,000—by four meals a day to get 500 calories per meal. Then, because according to the National Heart, Lung, and Blood Institute, you should get no more than 60 percent of your calories from carbs, we kept each entrée's carbohydrates below 75 grams, each snack less than 30 grams, and each side dish less than 25 grams. But if you eat more than one dish per meal, take that into account. And be sure to coordinate your medicine with your meals.

CHICKEN AND TURKEY MAIN DISHES

BEEF AND PORK MAIN DISHES

BEVERAGES AND BREAKFASTS

Bring-on-the-Morning Smoothie

2 c blueberries, raspberries, and/or
    strawberries, hulled (may use frozen)

$^1/_2$ banana

$^1/_2$ c orange juice

$^1/_2$ c crushed ice

1 Tbsp lime juice

Mint leaves (optional)

In a blender, combine berries, banana, orange juice, ice, and lime juice and blend until smooth. Pour into 2 glasses and garnish with mint leaves, if using.

Makes 2 servings

Per serving: 120 cal, 2 g pro, 29 g carb, 1 g fat, 0 g sat fat, 0 mg chol, 9 g fiber, 4 mg sodium

Diet Exchanges: 0 milk, 0 vegetable, 2 fruit, 0 starch/bread, 0 meat, 0 fat

Frothy Hot Chocolate

Photo on page 279

1 c 1% milk

2 Tbsp unsweetened cocoa powder

2 Tbsp maple syrup

In small saucepan over medium heat, bring evaporated milk, cocoa, and maple syrup to a boil, whisking to prevent lumps.

Reduce heat to low. Cook 2 minutes, whisking constantly, until hot and frothy.

Makes 2 servings

Per serving: 116 cal, 5g pro, 22 g carb, 2 g fat, 1 g sat fat, 6 mg chol, 2 g fiber, 56 mg sodium

Diet Exchanges: 0.5 milk, 0 vegetable, 0 fruit, 1 starch/bread, 0 meat, 0 fat

Very Berry Parfait

$^3/_4$ c low-fat cottage cheese

3 Tbsp confectioners' sugar

2 tsp granulated sugar

$^1/_4$ tsp pure vanilla extract

4 c blueberries

4 tsp semisweet mini chocolate morsels

1. In a blender, combine cottage cheese, sugars, and vanilla extract. Blend on high until mixture is smooth and creamy.

2. Spoon $^1/_2$ cup berries into each of 4 parfait glasses. Spoon 2 heaping tablespoons cheese mixture on top of berries. Add another layer of $^1/_2$ cup berries. Top with 1 heaping tablespoon of cheese mixture. Sprinkle 1 teaspoon chocolate morsels on top of each parfait.

Makes 4 servings

Per serving: 160 cal, 5 g pro, 33 g carb, 3 g fat, 2 g sat fat, 5 mg chol, 4 g fiber, 150 mg sodium

Diet Exchanges: 0 milk, 0 vegetable, $1^1/_2$ fruit, 1 starch/bread, 1 meat, 0.5 fat

Fruit Salad

1 med blood orange, peeled and sectioned

1 med ruby red grapefruit, peeled and sectioned

Juice from $^1/_2$ med Valencia orange

8 fresh mint leaves

$^1/_4$ c whole pecans

$^1/_2$ tsp ground cinnamon

Place orange and grapefruit in large bowl. Add orange juice and toss to coat. Top with mint, pecans, and cinnamon.

Makes 5 servings

Per serving: 74 cal, 1 g pro, 9 g carb, 4 g fat, 0.5 g sat fat, 0 mg chol, 1 g fiber, 0 mg sodium

Diet Exchanges: 0 milk, 0.5 vegetable, 0 fruit, 0 starch/bread, 2 meat, 1 fat

Granola Pancakes with Fruit Sauce

Photo on page 280

Pancakes

1 c low-fat buttermilk

1 egg, at room temperature

3 Tbsp melted butter

$^3/_4$ c all-purpose flour

1 tsp baking soda

2 tsp sugar (optional)

$^1/_2$ c low-fat granola

Sauce

1 c fresh berries (whole or sliced)

1 Tbsp maple syrup

$^1/_2$ tsp freshly squeezed lemon juice

1. To prepare pancakes: In small bowl, combine buttermilk, egg, and melted butter. Stir until smooth. In medium bowl, combine flour, baking soda, and sugar, if using. Stir until well blended. Add liquid mix and stir until just blended.

2. To prepare sauce: In small saucepan, combine berries, maple syrup, and lemon juice. Cook over medium heat about 8 minutes or just until berries are soft and release their juices. Keep warm, if desired.

3. Heat lightly oiled skillet or griddle to medium high. Ladle 2 tablespoons of batter onto skillet. Sprinkle with 1 tablespoon granola. When little bubbles begin to form, flip pancake and cook 1 to 2 minutes on other side. Repeat with remaining batter and granola. Serve warm with fruit sauce and granola sprinkled on top, if desired.

Makes 4 servings

Per serving: (2 pancakes and 2 teaspoons sauce) 290 cal, 8 g pro, 40 g carb, 11 g fat, 6 g sat fat, 78 mg chol, 2 g fiber, 492 mg sodium

Diet Exchanges: 0 milk, 0 vegetable, 0.5 fruit, 2 starch/bread, 0 meat, 2 fat

Pepper Jack Frittata

1 red bell pepper, chopped

1 green bell pepper, chopped

$^3/_4$ c (3 oz) shredded pepper Jack cheese

15 flat-leaf parsley leaves, chopped

$1^3/_4$ c liquid egg substitute

Preheat oven to 375°F. Coat 9" nonstick pie pan with butter-flavored cooking spray. Sprinkle peppers, cheese, and parsley in pan. Pour in egg substitute. Bake 30 minutes. Cool slightly. Cut into wedges.

Makes 4 servings

Per serving: 150 cal, 16 g pro, 6 g carb, 7 g fat, 4 g sat fat, 20 mg chol, 1 g fiber, 380 mg sodium

Diet Exchanges: 0 milk, 0.5 vegetable, 0 fruit, 0 starch/bread, 2 meat, 1 fat

Four-Step Fontina Frittata

6 lg eggs

3 c Summer Squash Sauté (see page 299)

$^1/_2$ c grated Fontina cheese

1 tsp olive oil

1. Preheat broiler. Position rack second from top.

2. Beat eggs in large bowl. Fold in squash and cheese.

3. Heat oil 2 to 3 minutes in medium nonstick, broiler-safe skillet over medium heat, turning pan to coat. Add egg mixture and cook 3 minutes to set bottom. Reduce heat to medium-low and cook 3 to 5 minutes, lifting edges occasionally and tilting pan so uncooked egg mixture flows to bottom.

4. Broil 3 to 4 minutes or until frittata is browned and set. Serve warm or at room temperature.

Makes 6 servings

Per serving: 177 cal, 11 g pro, 7 g carb, 12.5 g fat, 4 g sat fat, 222 mg chol, 2 g fiber, 291 mg sodium

Diet Exchanges: 0 milk, 1 vegetable, 0 fruit, 0 starch/bread, 1 meat, 2 fat

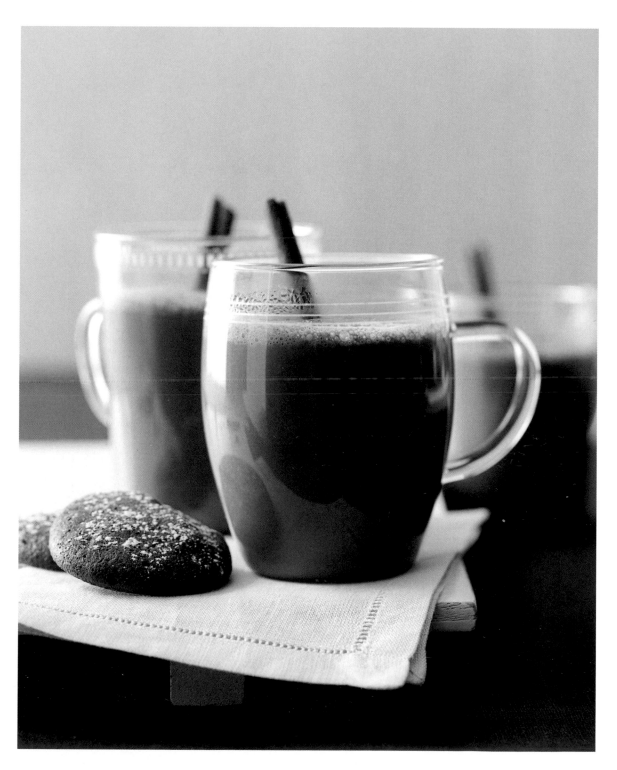

Frothy Hot Chocolate
Recipe on page 275

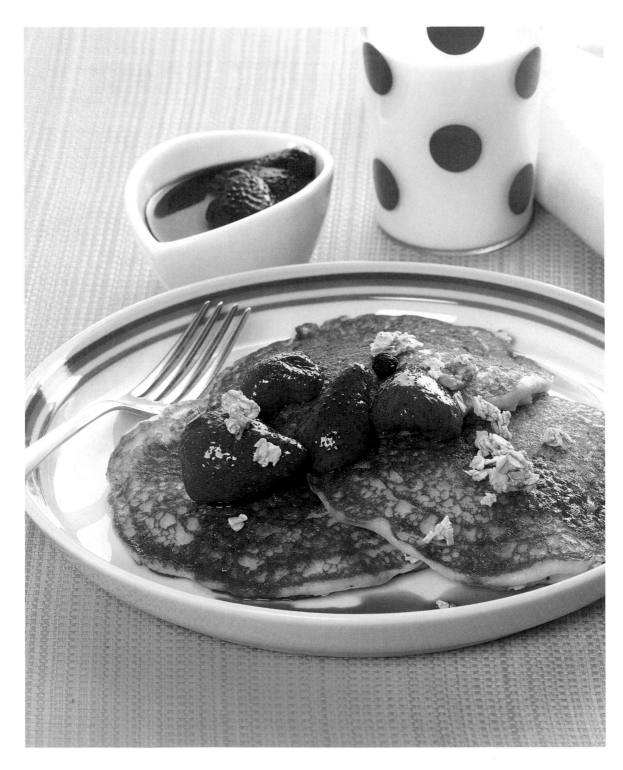

Granola Pancakes with Fruit Sauce
Recipe on page 277

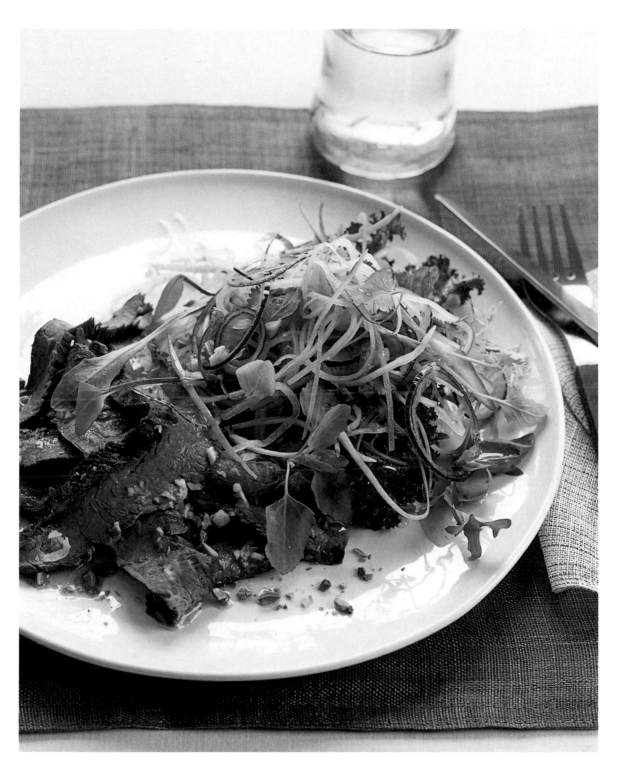

Vietnamese Beef Salad
Recipe on page 288

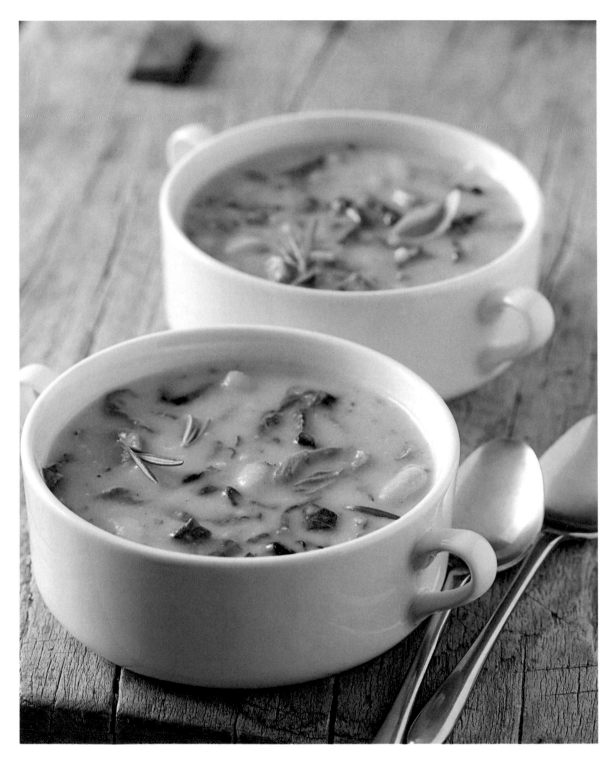

Creamy Roasted-Garlic Soup
Recipe on page 294

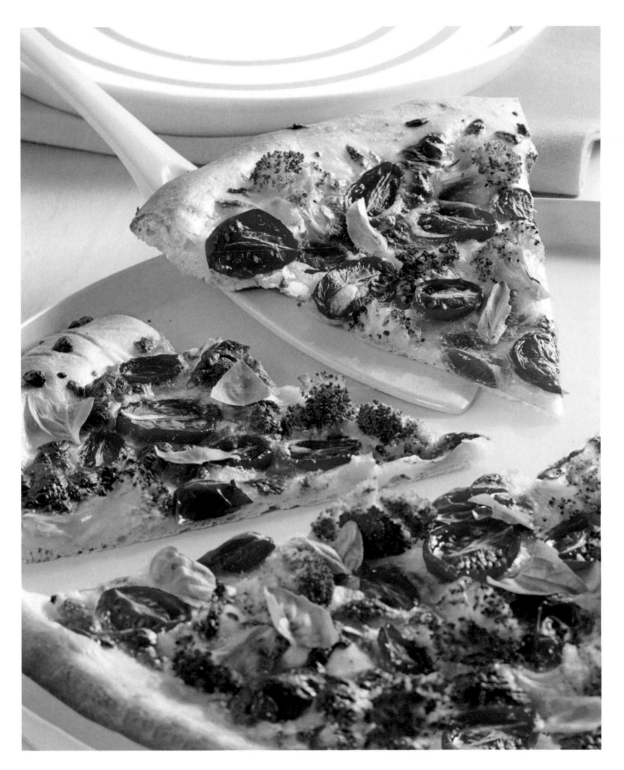

Tricolor Pizza
Recipe on page 302

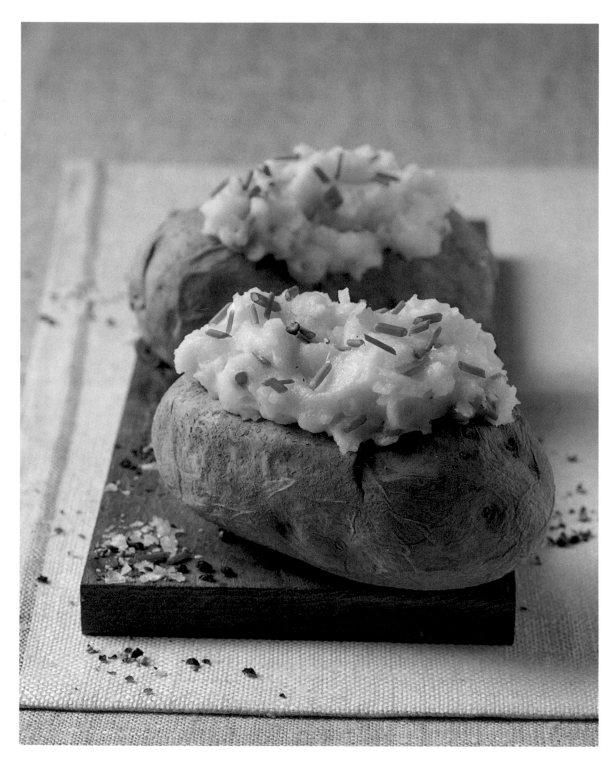

284 Healthier Twice-Baked Potatoes
Recipe on page 306

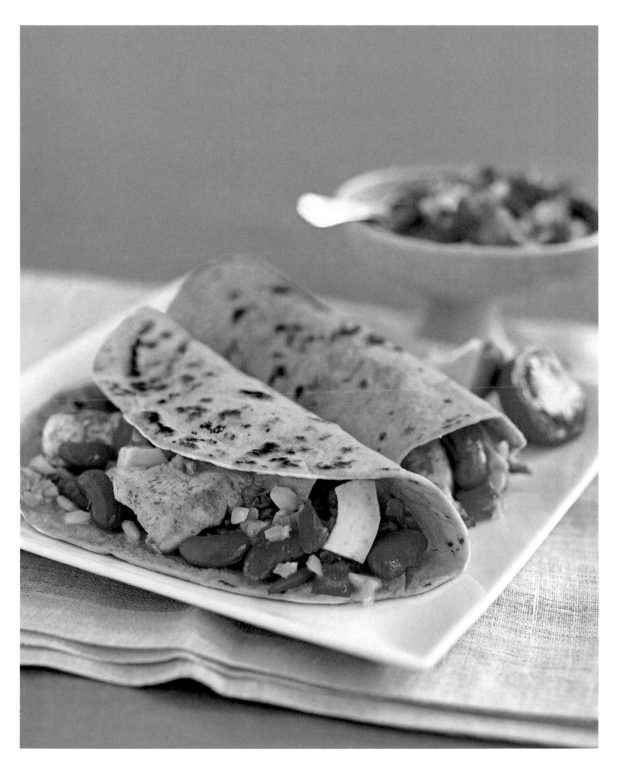

Soft Tacos with Chicken and Kidney Beans
Recipe on page 312

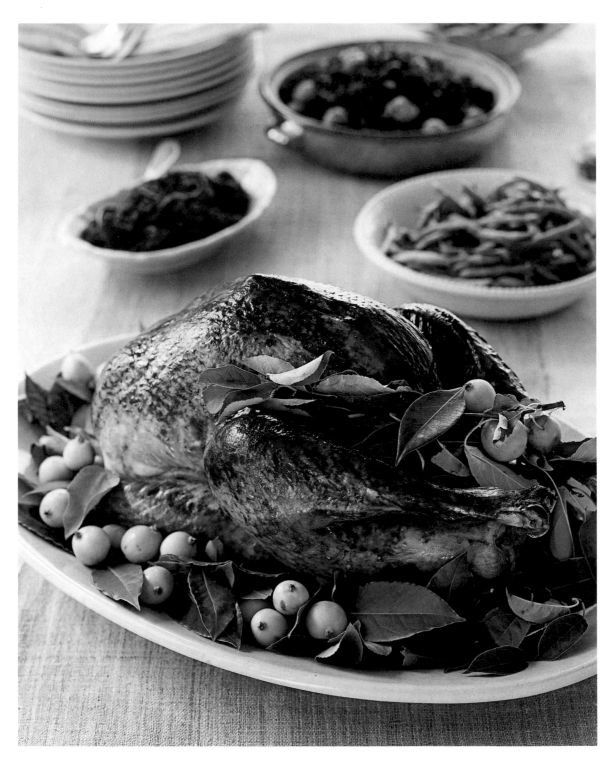

Roast Turkey with Apple and Orange Pan Juices
Recipe on page 324

Cardamom Biscuits

$1^1/_2$ c whole wheat flour

$1/_3$ c nonfat dry milk

2 tsp baking powder

$1/_4$ tsp (rounded) ground cardamom

$1/_8$ tsp salt

$1/_3$ c warm 2% milk

$1/_3$ c honey

3 Tbsp vegetable oil

$1/_2$ tsp pure vanilla extract

1 Tbsp coarse sugar

1. Preheat oven to 425°F. Lightly coat baking sheet with cooking spray.

2. Combine flour, dry milk, baking powder, cardamom, and salt in medium bowl. In separate medium bowl, blend milk, honey, oil, and vanilla extract. Stir in dry ingredients until just combined. (There will be some lumps in the loose dough.)

3. Knead briefly, until dough just comes together. Transfer dough onto lightly floured surface and pat into 9" × 3" rectangle.

4. Using long knife, divide rectangle into 3 squares. Then cut each square diagonally to make 6 triangles. Transfer to prepared baking sheet. Bake in center of oven 6 minutes. Sprinkle tops with sugar and bake 8 minutes more. Cool completely on rack.

Makes 6 biscuits

Per biscuit: 248 cal, 6 g pro, 42 g carb, 8 g fat, 1.5 g sat fat, 2 mg chol, 4 g fiber, 212 mg sodium

Diet Exchanges: 0 milk, 0 vegetable, 0 fruit, 2 starch/bread, 2 meat, 1.5 fat

SALADS AND SOUPS

Vietnamese Beef Salad

Photo on page 281

¼ c reduced-sodium soy sauce

¼ c freshly squeezed lime juice

¼ c water

2 Tbsp sugar

1 Tbsp minced garlic

2 tsp chile paste

½ lb flank steak

6 c mixed greens

1 c sliced fresh basil

1 c chopped fresh cilantro

2 lg red onions, thinly sliced (about 2 c)

2 lg seedless cucumbers, with peel, julienned (about 4 c)

4 med carrots, julienned (about 2 c)

2 Tbsp chopped dry-roasted, unsalted peanuts

1. Whisk together soy sauce, lime juice, water, sugar, garlic, and chile paste in medium bowl. Pour 3 tablespoons into resealable plastic bag. Cover and chill remaining dressing for salad. Add steak to bag, seal, and turn to coat. Chill 30 minutes.

2. Heat grill or broiler to medium-high. Grill steak 8 to 10 minutes, turning once, for medium-rare. (Thermometer should register 145°F.) Let rest 5 minutes and slice thinly at an angle, across the grain.

3. Toss together greens, basil, and cilantro in large bowl. Evenly divide among 4 plates. Sprinkle with onions, cucumbers, and carrots. Top with steak, drizzle with dressing, and sprinkle with peanuts.

Makes 4 servings

Per serving: 260 cal, 18 g pro, 30 g carb, 8.5 g fat, 2.5 g sat fat, 24 mg chol, 6 g fiber, 660 mg sodium

Diet Exchanges: 0 milk, 3.5 vegetable, 0 fruit, 0.5 starch/bread, 2 meat, 0.5 fat

Crab Salad with Avocado and Pomelo

Dressing

2 Tbsp freshly squeezed orange juice

2 Tbsp white wine vinegar

1½ Tbsp extra-virgin olive oil

2 tsp finely chopped fresh tarragon or chervil

½ tsp freshly grated orange zest

½ tsp salt

¼ tsp dry mustard

¼ tsp freshly ground black pepper

Salad

2 heads butterhead lettuce, separated into leaves (about 8 c)

2 med sweet onions, sliced (about 2 c)

2 pomelos, peeled and cut into sections (about 4 c); substitute grapefruit if unavailable

1 med avocado, peeled, pitted, and sliced

1 c lump crabmeat (available at fish counter)

1 Tbsp chopped toasted skinless hazelnuts

1. To prepare dressing: Whisk together orange juice, vinegar, oil, tarragon, orange zest, salt, mustard, and pepper in medium bowl. Set aside.

2. To prepare salad: Combine lettuce, onions, and pomelos in large bowl. Toss with dressing and mound onto 4 plates. Fan out a quarter of the avocado on top of each and top with crabmeat and hazelnuts.

Makes 4 servings

Per serving: 285 cal, 11 g pro, 32 g carb, 15 g fat, 2 g sat fat, 30 mg chol, 8 g fiber, 335 mg sodium

Diet Exchanges: 0 milk, 1.5 vegetable, 0.5 fruit, 0 starch/bread, 1 meat, 3 fat

Italian Shrimp and Chickpea Salad

2 c canned chickpeas, rinsed and drained

1 lb med cooked, peeled, and deveined shrimp

2 med tomatoes (about $1/2$ lb), seeded and chopped

6 lg leaves basil, chopped

$1/4$ c olive oil

4 c arugula

In large bowl, gently toss chickpeas, shrimp, tomatoes, basil, and oil. Season with salt and freshly ground black pepper to taste. Serve over arugula.

Makes 6 servings

Per serving: 270 cal, 23 g pro, 21 g carb, 12 g fat, 1.5 g sat fat, 145 mg chol, 6 g fiber, 180 mg sodium

Diet Exchanges: 0 milk, 0.5 vegetable, 0 fruit, 1 starch/bread, 2.5 meat, 2 fat

Sugar Snap Peas and Fennel Salad with Apple Cider Vinaigrette

2 Tbsp apple cider vinegar

2 tsp honey

$^3/_4$ tsp Dijon mustard

$^1/_4$ tsp salt

$1^1/_2$ tsp extra-virgin olive oil

$^1/_4$ c grated sweet onion (such as Vidalia or Walla Walla)

1 Tbsp chopped fresh tarragon or other favorite herb

2 tsp finely chopped shallot

$2^1/_2$ c sugar snap peas, tough strings removed

$1^1/_2$ c shelled fresh peas

1 sm fennel bulb, trimmed, halved, and cut into bite-size strips

Whisk together vinegar, honey, mustard, and salt in medium bowl. Then whisk in oil. Stir in onion, tarragon, and shallot, and season with salt and freshly ground black pepper. Toss with snap peas, peas, and fennel.

Makes 6 servings

Per serving: 87 cal, 4 g pro, 15 g carb, 1.5 g fat, 0 g sat fat, 0 mg chol, 4 g fiber, 141 mg sodium

Diet Exchanges: 0 milk, 1.5 vegetable, 0 fruit, 0.5 starch/bread, 0 meat, 0 fat

Black-Eyed Peas and Vegetable Salad

1 med onion, quartered

1 med green or red bell pepper, cored and seeded

1 lg clove garlic

1 sm jalapeño chile pepper, cored and seeded (wear plastic gloves when handling)

2 c rinsed and drained canned black-eyed peas

$^1/_4$ c canola oil

3 Tbsp white vinegar

1. In food processor, finely chop onion, bell pepper, garlic, and jalapeño pepper until mixture is a fine mince but not a paste.

2. In large bowl, toss black-eyed peas and chopped vegetables. Add oil and vinegar and season with salt and freshly ground black pepper, if desired. Toss well to combine.

Makes 6 servings

Per serving: 159 cal, 4 g pro, 15 g carb, 10 g fat, 1 g sat fat, 0 mg chol, 3 g fiber, 241 mg sodium

Diet Exchanges: 0 milk, 0.5 vegetable, 0 fruit, 1 starch/bread, 0 meat, 2 fat

Curried Tofu with Asian Slaw

Marinade

¼ c light coconut milk

2 Tbsp curry powder

1 Tbsp minced garlic

1 Tbsp reduced-sodium soy sauce

1 container (14 oz) extra-firm tofu, drained,
   patted dry, and cut into ½"-thick,
   1" × 2" strips

Dressing

⅓ c rice wine vinegar

¼ c unsalted peanut butter

2 Tbsp reduced-sodium soy sauce

1 Tbsp freshly squeezed lime juice

1 Tbsp honey

2 tsp minced garlic

½ tsp red curry paste (sold in ethnic-food
   section of most supermarkets)

Salad

1 head napa cabbage, thinly sliced
   (about 6 c)

3 med red bell peppers, julienned
   (about 3 c)

6 med carrots, julienned (about 3 c)

1 c thinly sliced scallions

⅓ c chopped fresh cilantro

1. To prepare marinade: In small bowl, combine coconut milk, curry powder, garlic, and soy sauce. Place tofu in wide bowl, add marinade, and turn each piece to coat. Marinate at least ½ hour and up to 4 (cover and chill in refrigerator if more than 2 hours).

2. Preheat broiler. Arrange tofu slices in single layer on foil-lined baking sheet. Coat lightly with cooking spray and broil 4 minutes. Gently turn tofu, coat lightly with spray, and broil 4 minutes longer or until golden brown. Remove from broiler and cool slightly.

3. To prepare dressing: In medium bowl, whisk together vinegar, peanut butter, soy sauce, lime juice, honey, garlic, and curry paste.

4. To prepare salad: In large bowl, combine cabbage, peppers, carrots, scallions, tofu, and half of the cilantro. Add dressing and toss well to coat. Divide among 4 bowls and top with remaining cilantro.

Makes 4 servings

Per serving: 340 cal, 19 g pro, 34 g carb, 16 g fat, 3 g sat fat, 0 mg chol, 8 g fiber, 670 mg sodium

Diet Exchanges: 0 milk, 3 vegetable, 0 fruit, 1 starch/bread, 2.5 meat, 3 fat

Cucumber and Melon Salad with Watercress, Herbs, and Feta

Dressing

2 Tbsp extra-virgin olive oil

2 Tbsp freshly squeezed lemon juice

2 Tbsp white wine vinegar

1 Tbsp minced shallot

1 tsp sugar

$^{1}/_{2}$ tsp salt

$^{1}/_{2}$ tsp freshly ground black pepper

Salad

8 c melon balls (1 honeydew or various types)

3 cucumbers, peeled and chopped (about 6 c)

1 bunch watercress (about 4 c)

$^{1}/_{2}$ c fresh mint leaves

$^{1}/_{2}$ c feta cheese

1 Tbsp toasted pine nuts

1 Tbsp kalamata olives, pitted and quartered lengthwise

1. To prepare dressing: Whisk together oil, lemon juice, vinegar, shallot, sugar, salt, and pepper in small bowl.

2. To prepare salad: Combine melon, cucumbers, watercress, and mint in large bowl. Toss with dressing, cheese, pine nuts, and olives.

Makes 4 servings

Per serving: 295 cal, 7 g pro, 41 g carb, 13.5 g fat, 4 g sat fat, 17 mg chol, 5 g fiber, 548 mg sodium

Diet Exchanges: 0 milk, 1 vegetable, 2 fruit, 0 starch/bread, 0.5 meat, 2.5 fat

Spaghetti Squash Salad with Honey-Ginger Chicken and Blue Cheese

1 lg spaghetti squash (about 4 lb)

1 Tbsp molasses

2 tsp minced garlic

2 tsp finely chopped fresh ginger

$^{1}/_{4}$ c honey, divided

$^{1}/_{4}$ c + 3 Tbsp balsamic vinegar, divided

2 lg boneless, skinless chicken breast halves (about 1 lb)

$^{1}/_{2}$ tsp salt

$^{1}/_{4}$ tsp freshly ground black pepper

1 tsp + 2 Tbsp extra-virgin olive oil, divided

3 Tbsp freshly squeezed orange juice

1 Tbsp minced shallot

2 Tbsp crumbled blue cheese

4 c arugula

1. Prick squash all over with fork or sharp knife. Microwave on high

8 minutes, turn over, and microwave another 8 minutes. When cool enough to handle, halve squash and scrape out seeds with spoon. Drag tines of fork along flesh to tease it into long, spaghetti-like strands. (You should have roughly 8 cups.) Spin squash in salad spinner to remove excess liquid. Cover and chill in refrigerator.

2. Whisk together molasses, garlic, ginger, 3 tablespoons of the honey, and $1/4$ cup of the vinegar in small bowl. Season chicken with salt and pepper. Heat 1 teaspoon of the oil in 10" non-stick skillet over medium-high heat. Sear chicken 6 minutes, flipping once. Add honey mixture to skillet. Reduce heat to medium-low and simmer 10 minutes or until thermometer inserted in thickest portion of chicken registers 160°F and juices run clear. Remove chicken and let cool. Shred chicken.

3. Combine orange juice, shallot, and remaining honey, vinegar, and oil in large bowl and stir well to emulsify oil and vinegar. Add chicken and blue cheese and toss to coat. Serve over squash and arugula.

Makes 4 servings

Per serving: 415 cal, 30 g pro, 48 g carb, 12 g fat, 2.5 g sat fat, 69 mg chol, 5 g fiber, 446 mg sodium

Diet Exchanges: 0 milk, 4.5 vegetable, 0 fruit, 1.5 starch/bread, 4 meat, 2 fat

Chicken and Rice Gumbo

1 lb boneless, skinless chicken breasts, cut into bite-size pieces

3 cans ($14 1/2$ oz each) reduced-sodium chicken broth

1 can ($14 1/2$ oz) no-salt-added stewed tomatoes, chopped

1 can (15 oz) whole-kernel corn, drained

$1/2$ tsp hot-pepper sauce

$1/2$ c quick-cooking rice

1. Place chicken in large pot. Add broth, tomatoes (with juice), corn, and hot-pepper sauce. Bring to a boil.

2. Reduce heat, cover, and simmer 15 minutes. Stir in rice and simmer 5 minutes or until chicken is no longer pink.

Makes 10 servings

Per serving: 107 cal, 13 g pro, 10 g carb, 1 g fat, 0 g sat fat, 26 mg chol, 1 g fiber, 426 mg sodium

Diet Exchanges: 0 milk, 0.5 vegetable, 0 fruit, 0.5 starch/bread, 2 meat, 0 fat

Spiced Cauliflower Soup

1 tsp canola oil

2 cinnamon sticks

2 tsp mild curry powder

1 med onion, halved and sliced

2 cloves garlic, minced

2 Tbsp water

3 c vegetable broth

$\frac{1}{2}$ head cauliflower, cut into sm florets

1 c thinly sliced mustard greens

1. Warm oil in large saucepan over medium heat. Add cinnamon sticks and cook about 2 minutes or until they are fragrant and begin to unfurl. Stir in curry powder and reduce heat to medium-low. Add onion, garlic, and water. Cook, stirring occasionally, 8 minutes or until onion is soft and translucent.

2. Add broth and cauliflower. Bring to a boil. Reduce heat and simmer, covered, 25 minutes or until cooked through.

3. Stir in mustard greens and cook until wilted, about 30 seconds. Discard cinnamon sticks.

Makes 4 servings

Per serving: 90 cal, 5 g pro, 14 g carb, 2 g fat, 0 g sat fat, 0 mg chol, 6 g fiber, 256 mg sodium

Diet Exchanges: 0 milk, 3 vegetable, 0 fruit, 0 starch/bread, 0 meat, 1.5 fat

Creamy Roasted-Garlic Soup

Photo on page 282

1 head garlic, unpeeled

1 Tbsp olive oil

1 lg yellow onion, chopped

1 container (32 oz) fat-free reduced-sodium chicken broth

$1\frac{1}{2}$ c leftover Smashed New Potatoes (about $\frac{1}{3}$ recipe see page 304)

2 c thinly sliced carrots

1 Tbsp chopped fresh rosemary

1 tsp dried basil

1 lg bunch Swiss chard, stemmed and chopped (about 8 c)

1 can (15 oz) cannellini beans, rinsed and drained

1. Preheat oven to 425°F. Slice off top third of garlic and discard. Wrap garlic in foil and roast 40 minutes. Let cool. Squeeze roasted garlic from papery skin into small bowl and discard skin.

2. Heat oil in large saucepan over medium-high heat. Add onion and cook

5 minutes or until translucent. Add broth and one-third of the garlic. Bring to a boil, reduce heat, and simmer 5 minutes.

3. Working in 2 batches, puree potatoes and onion-broth mixture together in blender until smooth. Return to pan.

4. Stir in carrots, rosemary, basil, and remaining garlic and cook over medium heat 10 minutes, stirring often.

5. Add chard, return to a simmer, and cook, stirring, 5 minutes. Add beans and cook 5 minutes longer.

Makes 8 servings

Per serving: 130 cal, 5 g pro, 23 g carb, 3 g fat, 0.5 g sat fat, 0 mg chol, 4 g fiber, 500 mg sodium

Diet Exchanges: 0 milk, 1.5 vegetable, 0 fruit, 1 starch/bread, 0 meat, 0.5 fat

Hearty Beef-Vegetable Soup

$^1/_2$ med onion, chopped

1 Tbsp vegetable oil

1 c canned salt free diced tomatoes

1 c frozen mixed vegetables

4 oz cooked beef, cubed or thinly sliced

$^3/_4$ tsp low-sodium beef base

4 c water

In medium saucepan, sauté onion in oil over medium-high heat 3 minutes. Add tomatoes, frozen vegetables, beef, beef base, and water. Simmer about 12 minutes or until vegetables are tender. Season to taste with salt and black pepper.

Makes 4 servings

Per serving: 180 cal, 8 g pro, 7 g carb, 12.5 g fat, 4 g sat fat, 25 mg chol, 2 g fiber, 136 mg sodium

Diet Exchanges: 0 milk, 1.5 vegetable, 0 fruit, 0 starch/bread, 1 meat, 2 fat

Asian Soup with Shrimp Dumplings

4 cloves garlic, smashed, divided

$1/2$" piece fresh ginger, peeled and smashed, divided

$1/2$ lb med shrimp, peeled (tails removed) and deveined

$1/4$ c cilantro leaves

2 tsp cornstarch

2 Tbsp water

1 Tbsp reduced-sodium soy sauce

$1/2$ tsp toasted sesame oil

6 c reduced-sodium chicken broth

1 stalk lemongrass, smashed and tied in knot, or $1/2$ tablespoon freshly grated lemon zest

$1/2$ tsp red-pepper flakes

1 c Garlicky Sautéed Greens (see page 310)

1. Mince half of the garlic and ginger in food processor. Add shrimp and cilantro and pulse to combine.

2. In small bowl, dissolve cornstarch in water. Add to shrimp with soy sauce and oil. Pulse to combine. Set aside.

3. Combine broth, lemongrass, red-pepper flakes, and remaining garlic and ginger in large saucepan over high heat. Bring to a boil. Reduce heat to low and let simmer.

4. Moisten hands and roll shrimp mixture into 12 balls while soup heats. When soup is simmering, drop in dumplings, one at a time. Simmer 6 to 7 minutes. Remove lemongrass. Divide greens evenly among 4 soup bowls, and ladle soup and 3 dumplings on top of each.

Makes 4 servings

Per serving: 158 cal, 20 g pro, 9 g carb, 5.5 g fat, 1 g sat fat, 111 mg chol, 1 g fiber, 507 mg sodium

Diet Exchanges: 0 milk, 0.5 vegetable, 0 fruit, 0.5 starch/bread, 2.5 meat, 0.5 fat

Middle Eastern Red Lentil Soup

1 Tbsp olive oil

1 med onion, finely chopped

2 med carrots, finely chopped

1 rib celery, finely chopped

1 c dried red lentils

2 Tbsp tomato paste

1/2 tsp ground cumin

1/4 tsp ground red pepper

5 c reduced-sodium chicken broth

6 Tbsp low-fat plain yogurt

1. Heat oil in medium soup pot over medium-high heat. Add onion, carrots, and celery and cook, stirring frequently, about 3 minutes or until vegetables begin to soften.

2. Stir in lentils, tomato paste, cumin, pepper, and broth. Raise heat to high and bring to a boil. Reduce heat and simmer, uncovered, stirring occasionally, 30 minutes or until lentils are soft and soup is thick. Salt to taste.

3. Place 1 cup of soup in food processor or blender. Puree until smooth. Combine with soup in pot and heat through.

4. Ladle into 6 preheated bowls and top each with 1 tablespoon of the yogurt.

Makes 6 servings

Per serving: 200 cal, 14 g pro, 27 g carb, 4.5 g fat, 1 g sat fat, 0 mg chol, 6 g fiber, 141 mg sodium

Diet Exchanges: 0 milk, 1 vegetable, 0 fruit, 1.5 starch/bread, 1 meat, 0.5 fat

VEGETARIAN AND SIDE DISHES

Love-Your-Broccoli Pasta

1 Tbsp olive oil

1 Tbsp minced fresh garlic

2 cans (14.5 oz each) seasoned diced
    tomatoes

1 Tbsp balsamic vinegar

1 tsp dried basil

$1/4$ tsp crushed red-pepper flakes

10 oz rigatoni

$1/2$ lb broccoli florets

$1/3$ c crumbled reduced-fat feta cheese

1. Bring large pot of salted water to a boil.

2. Heat oil in large skillet over medium-low heat. Add garlic and cook gently 1 minute. Add tomatoes (with juice), vinegar, basil, and red-pepper flakes. Increase heat and bring sauce to a simmer. Cook 15 minutes, stirring frequently.

3. While sauce is simmering, add rigatoni to the boiling water. When pasta is almost done, add broccoli to pot and cook 2 minutes longer.

4. Drain pasta and broccoli and transfer to large bowl. Add sauce and toss well. Sprinkle with cheese.

Makes 4 servings

Per serving: 364 cal, 15 g pro, 65 g carb, 7 g fat, 1.5 g sat fat, 5 mg chol, 5 g fiber, 671 mg sodium

Diet Exchanges: 0 milk, 2 vegetable, 0 fruit, 3 starch/bread, 0.5 meat, 1 fat

In-a-Jiffy Pasta with Marinara

2 tsp olive oil

1 med onion, chopped

1 clove garlic, crushed

1 can (28 oz) diced tomatoes

2 tsp tomato paste

$1/4$ tsp dried oregano

8 cups cooked spaghetti squash (yield from
    a 4-pound squash)

1. Heat oil in medium saucepan over medium heat. Once hot, add onion and sauté 3 minutes or until softened. Toss in garlic and cook 2 minutes. Stir in tomatoes (with juice), tomato paste, and oregano. Simmer, uncovered, about 25 minutes.

2. While sauce is simmering, prepare squash. Pierce skin with a fork in several times. Place in a 350°F oven on a baking sheet for 25 to 30 minutes, or

until skin is tender. Remove from oven and allow to cool slightly. Cut squash in half lengthwise and scoop out seeds. Using a fork, pull apart strands of the hot squash and place in a serving bowl.

Makes 4 servings

Per serving: 158 cal, 4 g pro, 29 g carb, 3 g fat, 0.5 g sat fat, 0 mg chol, 6 g fiber, 543 mg sodium

Diet Exchanges: 0 milk, 6 vegetable, 0 fruit, 0 starch/bread, 0 meat, 0.5 fat

Zucchini Rotini

$1/4$ c whole wheat rotini (or other pasta)

1 c fat-free cottage cheese

1 Tbsp salt-free Italian seasoning

$1/2$ c shredded zucchini

1 c canned diced tomatoes, drained

$1/2$ c reduced-fat shredded mozzarella cheese

1. Prepare rotini per package directions. Drain and set aside.

2. In small baking dish, combine cottage cheese and Italian seasoning. Stir in reserved rotini and zucchini. Top with tomatoes and sprinkle with mozzarella. Microwave on high 3 minutes to warm through, or broil about 5 minutes or until bubbly.

Makes 2 servings

Per serving: 227 cal, 23 g pro, 25 g carb, 4.7 g fat, 3 g sat fat, 23 mg chol, 4 g fiber, 768 mg sodium

Diet Exchanges: 0 milk, 1 vegetable, 0 fruit, 0.5 starch/bread, 3 meat, 0.5 fat

Summer Squash Sauté

6 cloves garlic, sliced

2 Tbsp extra-virgin olive oil

1 tsp red-pepper flakes

3 lb assorted summer squash (zucchini, yellow crookneck, etc.), thinly sliced

$1/2$ tsp salt

Heat garlic, oil, and red-pepper flakes in large sauté pan over medium heat 2 to 3 minutes or until garlic begins to turn golden. Add squash and salt. Toss to coat. Cover, reduce heat to medium-low, and cook 30 minutes, stirring occasionally, until squash begins to break apart. Uncover, increase heat to medium, and cook 10 to 12 minutes longer or until liquid is almost gone.

Makes 8 servings

Per serving: 61 cal, 2 g pro, 6 g carb, 4 g fat, 0.5 g sat fat, 0 mg chol, 2 g fiber, 149 mg sodium

Diet Exchanges: 0 milk, 1 vegetable, 0 fruit, 0 starch/bread, 0 meat, 1 fat

Macaroni and Cheese

$1/2$ lb whole wheat elbow macaroni

$1/4$ c all-purpose flour

$1/2$ tsp mustard powder

$2^1/2$ c 1% milk

$1^1/2$ c shredded reduced-fat, extra sharp
Cheddar cheese

2 Tbsp dried bread crumbs

1. Preheat oven to 350°F. Coat $2^1/2$-quart baking dish with cooking spray.

2. Prepare macaroni per package directions and drain.

3. Place flour and mustard in medium saucepan. Gradually add milk, whisking constantly, until smooth. Place over medium heat. Cook, whisking constantly, 8 minutes or until thickened. Remove from heat. Stir in cheese until smooth. Stir in macaroni and place in baking dish.

4. Sprinkle bread crumbs over macaroni. Bake 20 minutes or until heated through.

Makes 6 servings

Per serving: 290 cal, 17 g pro, 40 g carb, 8 g fat, 5 g sat fat, 25 mg chol, 3 g fiber, 310 mg sodium

Diet Exchanges: 0.5 milk, 0 vegetable, 0 fruit, 2 starch/bread, 1 meat, 1 fat

Toasted Vegetable Taco

1–2 c chopped mixed fresh vegetables, such
as broccoli, snap peas, green beans,
and red bell pepper

4 flour tortilla (8" diameter)

1.5 Tbsp prepared raspberry chipotle sauce

$1/4$ c shredded taco-cheese mix

1. Place vegetables in microwaveable bowl. Cover with plastic wrap and microwave on high 3–4 minutes or until crisp-tender.

2. Bend each tortilla until edges meet, but do not fold. Carefully toast in a toaster.

3. Spread sauce on each tortilla. Top each with vegetables and sprinkle with cheese.

Makes 4 serving

Per serving: 190 cal, 7 g pro, 30 g carb, 6 g fat, 2 g sat fat, 5 mg chol, 3 g fiber, 368 mg sodium

Diet Exchanges: 0 milk 0.5 vegetable, 0 fruit, 1.5 starch/bread, 0 meat, 0.5 fat

Veggie Pizza

4 English muffin, split

1 c tomato sauce

1 c chopped mushrooms

$^1/_2$ c chopped green bell pepper

$^1/_2$ c chopped onion

$^1/_2$ c shredded reduced-fat mozzarella
cheese

1. Preheat oven or toaster oven to 350°F.

2. Toast muffin halves. Evenly divide
sauce, mushrooms, bell pepper, onion,
and cheese between muffin halves.

3. Place muffin halves on a large
baking sheet. Bake 3 minutes or until
cheese is melted.

Makes 4 serving

Per serving: 206 cal, 11 g pro, 34 g carb, 3.5 g fat,
1.5 g sat fat, 8 mg chol, 3 g fiber, 671 mg sodium

Diet Exchanges: 0 milk, 1 vegetable, 0 fruit,
2 starch/bread, 0.5 meat, 0 fat

Greek Pizza

$^1/_2$ c dry-packed sun-dried tomatoes

1 Tbsp freshly squeezed lemon juice

2 c Garlicky Sautéed Greens (see page 310)

1 whole wheat pizza crust (12" diameter; we
used thin-crust Boboli)

5 kalamata olives, pitted and chopped

3 oz mild feta cheese, crumbled (we used
Athenos)

2 tsp fresh oregano leaves

1. Preheat oven to 400°F, preferably
with a pizza stone inside. Meanwhile,
soak tomatoes in hot water 10 minutes
or until soft. Drain and chop.

2. Squeeze lemon juice onto greens and
then scatter greens onto pizza crust.
Top with tomatoes and olives, crumble
feta on top, and sprinkle with oregano.

3. Bake 12 minutes, directly on rack or
pizza stone, or until cheese is soft and
golden in spots and crust is crisp.

Makes 8 servings

Per serving: 162 cal, 8 g pro, 21 g carb, 7 g fat, 2 g
sat fat, 6 mg chol, 4 g fiber, 502 mg sodium

Diet Exchanges: 0 milk, 1 vegetable, 0 fruit,
0 starch/bread, 0 meat, 0.5 fat

Tricolor Pizza

Photo on page 283

1 head broccoli, separated into small florets

2 prebaked regular or whole wheat pizza
    shells (12" diameter), such as Boboli

1 c reduced-fat shredded mozzarella cheese

1 pt cherry tomatoes, halved

6 Tbsp grated Parmesan cheese

1 c torn basil leaves (optional)

1. Preheat oven to 500°F.

2. In large pot of rapidly boiling water, cook broccoli, uncovered, 2 minutes or until crisp-tender. Drain and set aside.

3. Place each pizza shell on baking sheet. Sprinkle with mozzarella, add an even layer of tomatoes, and dot with broccoli. Place in oven and bake about 8 minutes or until crusts are golden brown and crisp. Remove from oven and sprinkle with Parmesan. Scatter pizzas with basil leaves, if desired. Cut each pie into six slices and serve.

Makes 6 servings

Per serving: 425 cal, 23 g pro, 53 g carb, 14 g fat, 6 g sat fat, 26 mg chol, 4 g fiber, 820 mg sodium

Diet Exchanges: 0 milk, 1 vegetable, 0 fruit, 0 starch/bread, 1.5 meat, 1 fat

Wild Rice, Almond, and Cranberry Dressing

2 c wild rice

1 rib celery, with leafy top

2 strips (2" × $1/2$") orange zest

2 tsp salt

6 c water

2 whole cloves

$1/2$ sm onion + 2 c chopped onion

1 Tbsp olive oil

2 cloves garlic, minced

2 c seedless green grapes

1 c dried cranberries

1 c fat-free chicken broth

$1/2$ c chopped Italian parsley

$1/2$ c sliced almonds, toasted

1. Preheat oven to 400°F.

2. Combine rice, celery, orange zest, salt, and water in deep, wide, 5-quart pot. Heat to a boil over high heat. Stick cloves into onion half and add to pan. Cook, covered, over medium-low heat 35 to 45 minutes or until rice is tender. Remove from heat and let stand, covered, 10 minutes. Discard orange zest, onion with cloves, and celery. Drain excess water if necessary. Set rice aside in pan.

3. Heat oil in large skillet over medium heat. Add chopped onion and stir to combine. Cover and cook over low heat about 5 minutes or until onions wilt. Cook, uncovered, over medium heat, stirring occasionally, about 10 minutes or until onions are golden. Add garlic and cook 1 minute.

4. Add onion-garlic mixture, grapes, cranberries, broth, and parsley to rice and stir to blend. Cover and cook over low heat 15 minutes. Spoon into 3-quart baking dish.

5. Bake for 55 minutes or until heated through. Uncover and sprinkle with almonds.

Makes 8 servings

Per serving: 164 cal, 5 g pro, 29 g carb, 5 g fat, 0.5 g sat fat, 0 mg chol, 5 g fiber, 650 mg sodium

Diet Exchanges: 0 milk, 0.5 vegetable, 0.5 fruit, 1 starch/bread, 0 meat, 0.5 fat

Sweet 'n' Tangy Carrots

2 c baby carrots

2 Tbsp honey

2 Tbsp Dijon mustard

Microwave carrots on high in 1 cup water for 5 minutes, then drain. Stir in honey and mustard while carrots are hot.

Makes 4 servings

Per serving: 67 cal, 1 g pro, 16 g carb, 0 g fat, 0 g sat fat, 0 mg chol, 1 g fiber, 218 mg sodium

Diet Exchanges: 0 milk, 1 vegetable, 0 fruit, 0.5 starch/bread, 0 meat, 0 fat

Potato Casserole

3 med potatoes, peeled and sliced

$\frac{1}{2}$ sm head cauliflower, coarsely chopped

1 tsp olive oil

1 med onion, chopped

2 oz veggie soy bacon, chopped

1 c shredded reduced-fat Cheddar cheese (4 oz)

1. Preheat oven to 350°F.

2. Bring large saucepan of water to a boil over medium-high heat. Add potatoes and boil 15 minutes or until fork-tender. Place in bowl with cauliflower. Mash with potato masher or electric mixer on medium speed.

3. Heat oil in small skillet over medium-high heat. Add onion and bacon and cook, stirring, 5 minutes or until soft.

4. Spoon half of potato mixture into baking dish. Sprinkle with half of the cheese and half of the onion-bacon mixture. Repeat layering to use remaining ingredients, ending with onion-bacon mixture.

5. Bake 10 minutes or until heated through and cheese has melted.

Makes 4 servings

Per serving: 210 cal, 14 g pro, 26 g carb, 7 g fat, 4 g sat fat, 20 mg chol, 4 g fiber, 330 mg sodium

Diet Exchanges: 0 milk, 1 vegetable, 0 fruit, 1$\frac{1}{2}$ starch/bread, 1 meat, 1 fat

Smashed New Potatoes

1$\frac{1}{2}$ lb sm new red potatoes, halved

$\frac{1}{4}$ c fat-free half-and-half

3 Tbsp fat-free sour cream

1 Tbsp unsalted butter

$\frac{1}{2}$ tsp salt

$\frac{1}{4}$ c fat-free milk

1. Place potatoes in medium saucepan and cover with cold water. Bring to a boil, reduce heat to a gentle boil, and cook 15 minutes or until tender. Drain and return to pan.

2. Briefly mash potatoes until broken up. Fold in half-and-half, sour cream, butter, salt, and enough milk to reach desired consistency.

Makes 8 servings

Per serving: 85 cal, 2 g pro, 15 g carb, 1.5 g fat, 1 g sat fat, 5 mg chol, 1 g fiber, 170 mg sodium

Diet Exchanges: 0 milk, 0 vegetable, 0 fruit, 1 starch/bread, 0 meat, 0.5 fat

Potato Pancakes over Baby Greens

2 c leftover Smashed New Potatoes
($1/2$ recipe; see opposite page)

$1/2$ c liquid egg substitute

$1/4$ c finely chopped onion

$1/4$ tsp red-pepper flakes

8 c baby greens

1 Tbsp white wine vinegar

1 Tbsp olive oil

$1/2$ tsp grainy Dijon mustard

$1/2$ c cherry tomatoes, halved

$1/4$ c freshly grated sharp Cheddar cheese

1. In large bowl, combine potatoes, egg substitute, onion, and red-pepper flakes.

2. Coat large nonstick skillet or griddle with cooking spray and heat to medium-high. Spoon $1/4$ cup mound of potato mixture onto hot pan. Repeat with 7 more mounds. Cook 15 minutes, turning once halfway through, until golden brown. (You may need to do this in batches, depending on the size of your skillet. Recoat pan with cooking spray in between batches.) Transfer to plate and keep warm.

3. Evenly divide greens among 4 serving plates.

4. In medium bowl, whisk vinegar, oil, and mustard. Add tomatoes. Drizzle over greens. Top each plate with 2 pancakes and sprinkle with cheese.

Makes 4 servings

Per serving: 195 cal, 10 g pro, 21 g carb, 9 g fat, 3 g sat fat, 13 mg chol, 4 g fiber, 314 mg sodium

Diet Exchanges: 0 milk, 1 vegetable, 0 fruit, 1 starch/bread, 1 meat, 1.5 fat

Healthier Twice-Baked Potatoes

Photo on page 284

4 med baking potatoes (6 oz each),
    scrubbed and pierced with fork

$^3/_4$ c shredded reduced-fat Cheddar cheese

4 Tbsp fat-free milk

1 scallion, finely chopped

5 tsp light butter, melted

4 tsp finely chopped fresh chives

1. Preheat oven to 400°F.

2. Place potatoes on baking sheet. Bake
50 to 60 minutes or until tender. Cool
10 minutes.

3. Cut each potato in half lengthwise.
Carefully scoop pulp from all pieces,
leaving shells of potatoes intact.

4. Add pulp, cheese, milk, scallion, and
3 teaspoons of the melted butter to
medium mixing bowl. Beat with
electric mixer until fluffy. Season with
salt and pepper to taste. Scoop filling
back into potato shells. Drizzle remaining 2 teaspoons butter evenly over tops.

5. Coat medium baking pan with olive
oil spray. Place potatoes in pan and

bake 10 to 15 minutes or until heated
through. Sprinkle with chives.

Makes 8 servings

Per serving: 115 cal, 5 g pro, 19 g carb, 2.2 g fat,
1.3 g sat fat, 5 mg chol, 2 g fiber, 95 mg sodium

Diet Exchanges: 0 milk, 0 vegetable, 0 fruit,
1 starch/bread, 1 meat, 0.5 fat

Mini Sweet-Potato Casseroles

$1^1/_2$ lb sweet potatoes, peeled and cut into
    $^1/_2$" cubes

$^1/_3$ c orange juice

$3^1/_2$ Tbsp light butter, melted

2 Tbsp fat-free half-and-half

$^1/_2$ tsp pumpkin pie spice

$^1/_8$ tsp salt

$^1/_8$ tsp black pepper

2 Tbsp finely chopped walnuts

1. Preheat oven to 400°F.

2. Place sweet potatoes in medium pot
and fill with enough cool water to cover.
Bring to a boil. Cover and cook until
very tender, about 10 minutes. Drain
potatoes and place in medium mixing
bowl. Add orange juice, butter, half-

and-half, and pumpkin pie spice. With electric hand mixer, beat mixture until smooth. Add salt and pepper.

3. Divide mixture among six 4-ounce ramekins and sprinkle 1 teaspoon of the walnuts over top of each. Bake 10 to 12 minutes or until walnuts are lightly toasted and tops of potatoes are lightly browned.

Makes 6 servings

Per serving: 148 cal, 2 g pro, 22 g carb, 6 g fat, 2.5 g sat fat, 10 mg chol, 3 g fiber, 144 mg sodium

Diet Exchanges: 0 milk, 0 vegetable, 0 fruit, 1 starch/bread, 0 meat, 1 fat

Roasted Rosemary Fingerlings

2 lb fingerling or tiny round potatoes (about 25), scrubbed and halved

2 tsp extra-virgin olive oil

$1^1/_2$ Tbsp minced garlic

$1^1/_2$ Tbsp chopped fresh rosemary

$^1/_4$ tsp salt

1. Preheat oven to 450°F.

2. Toss potatoes with oil, garlic, rosemary, and salt.

3. Place potatoes in single layer (so they don't touch) on nonstick baking sheet or in medium nonstick roasting pan. Roast 25 minutes or until tender inside, flipping potatoes and rotating pan occasionally to promote even browning.

Makes 6 servings

Per serving: 134 cal, 3 g pro, 27 g carb, 1.7 g fat, 0 g sat fat, 0 mg chol, 3 g fiber, 105 mg sodium

Diet Exchanges: 0 milk, 0 vegetable, 0 fruit, 1.5 starch/bread, 0 meat, 0.5 fat

Whipped Sweet and Yukon Gold Potatoes

2½ lb Yukon gold potatoes, peeled and cut
    into 1" chunks

8 cloves garlic, smashed

2 bay leaves

1 tsp salt

2½ lb sweet potatoes, peeled and cut into
    1" chunks

1 c fat-free milk

2 Tbsp unsalted butter, melted

2 Tbsp grated Parmesan cheese

1. Preheat oven to 400°F. Lightly coat 2-quart baking dish with cooking spray.

2. Combine Yukon gold potatoes, half of the garlic, and 1 bay leaf in 3-quart saucepan. Add water to cover and ½ teaspoon of the salt.

3. Combine sweet potatoes and remaining garlic and bay leaf in second saucepan. Add water to cover and remaining ½ teaspoon salt. Cover saucepans and bring to a boil over high heat. Reduce heat to medium-low and cook until potatoes are fork-tender, about 15 minutes. Set aside ½ cup of cooking water from each saucepan.

4. Drain potatoes and put in separate large mixing bowls. Set aside garlic with potatoes and discard bay leaves.

5. Whip potatoes in each bowl with electric mixer until smooth. Gradually beat ½ cup of the milk into each bowl until blended. Add up to ½ cup of the reserved cooking water to each bowl to achieve a smooth, fluffy texture.

6. Spoon Yukon gold potatoes in half of the dish and sweet potatoes in other half. Drizzle top with butter and sprinkle with cheese. Bake about 55 minutes or until heated through.

Makes 16 servings

Per serving: 143 cal, 3 g pro, 28 g carb, 3.5 g fat, 2 g sat fat, 5 mg chol, 3 g fiber, 176 mg sodium

Diet Exchanges: 0 milk, 0 vegetable, 0 fruit, 1 starch/bread, 0 meat, 0.5 fat

Ginger-and-Garlic Green Beans with Red Bell-Pepper Strips

2 pkg (12 oz) frozen cut green beans

1 Tbsp olive oil

1 c frozen red bell pepper strips

2 tsp minced garlic

2 tsp grated fresh ginger

1. Cook beans per package directions. Drain and rinse with cold water.

2. Warm large skillet over medium heat and add oil and peppers. Cook, stirring constantly, 3 minutes. Add garlic and ginger and stir 30 seconds. Add beans and cook, stirring constantly, 3 minutes until heated through. Add 2 tablespoons water, stir, and serve.

Makes 8 servings

Per serving: 50 cal, 1 g pro, 6 g carb, 1.5 g fat, 0 g sat fat, 0 mg chol, 2 g fiber, 0 mg sodium

Diet Exchanges: 0 milk, 1 vegetable, 0 fruit, 0 starch/bread, 0 meat, 0.5 fat

Grilled Corn with Lime and Red Pepper

4 ears corn, husked

$1/4$ tsp salt

$1/8$ tsp ground red pepper

1 lime, quartered lengthwise

1. Bring large pot of water to a boil and preheat grill to medium-high.

2. Boil corn 5 minutes and remove to plate. Coat lightly with olive oil spray and grill 10 minutes, turning every 2 minutes.

3. Combine salt and pepper in small bowl. When corn is done, rub each ear with lime wedge and sprinkle with salt-and-pepper mixture.

Makes 4 servings

Per serving: 80 cal, 3 g pro, 18 g carb, 1 g fat, 0 g sat fat, 0 mg chol, 2 g fiber, 160 mg sodium

Diet Exchanges: 0 milk, 0 vegetable, 0 fruit, 1 starch/bread, 0 meat, 0 fat

Garlicky Sautéed Greens

6 cloves garlic, sliced

2 Tbsp extra-virgin olive oil

16 c (packed) stemmed and roughly
   chopped Swiss chard (about 5 lg
   bunches)

$\frac{1}{2}$ tsp red-pepper flakes

$\frac{1}{2}$ tsp kosher salt

1. Heat garlic and oil in large skillet over medium-low heat until garlic begins to turn golden, about 3 minutes. Transfer mixture to small bowl and set aside.

2. Add greens, red-pepper flakes, and salt to skillet. Using tongs, turn greens until wilted enough to fit in pan. Raise heat to medium, cover, and cook 7 to 10 minutes, tossing occasionally. Transfer greens to a colander to drain. Return greens to pan and toss with reserved garlic and oil mixture. Refrigerate leftover greens in an airtight container for up to 3 days.

Makes 8 servings

Per serving: 49 cal, 1 g pro, 4 g carb, 4 g fat, 0.5 g sat fat, 0 mg chol, 1 g fiber, 274 mg sodium

Diet Exchanges: 0 milk, 0.5 vegetable, 0 fruit, 0 starch/bread, 0 meat, 1 fat

Grilled Endive

6 Belgian endives, halved lengthwise

2 Tbsp grapeseed oil or vegetable oil

4 med tomatoes, cored and sliced about
   $\frac{1}{4}$" thick

1. Heat grill to medium. Brush endives with oil and season lightly with salt and freshly ground black pepper. Grill 2 to 3 minutes, cut side down, or until slightly charred and softened.

2. Place endives on platter and arrange tomatoes alongside.

Makes 6 servings

Per serving 67 cal, 1 g pro, 6 g carb, 5 g fat, 0.5 g sat fat, 0 mg chol, 3 g fiber, 6 mg sodium

Diet Exchanges: 0 milk, 1 vegetable, 0 fruit, 0 starch/bread, 0 meat, 1 fat

Cilantro Rice

2½ c reduced-sodium vegetable broth or
    water

1½ c brown basmati rice

1½ Tbsp grapeseed oil or canola oil

½ tsp salt

1½ c chopped fresh cilantro

1 tsp freshly squeezed lemon juice

1. Combine broth or water, rice, and oil in medium saucepan and bring nearly to a boil over high heat. Reduce to a simmer, cover, and cook about 50 minutes or until liquid is absorbed and rice is tender. Remove from heat and let stand 10 minutes.

2. Season with salt and freshly ground black pepper to taste. Add cilantro and lemon juice and fluff rice with fork.

Makes 6 servings

Per serving: 156 cal, 3 g pro, 28 g carb, 5 g fat, 0.5 g sat fat, 0 mg chol, 2 g fiber, 333 mg sodium

Diet Exchanges: 0 milk, 0.5 vegetable, 0 fruit, 1.5 starch/bread, 0 meat, 1 fat

Cranberry-Orange Relish

1 sm unpeeled navel orange, cut into chunks

½ c pitted dried dates

1 lg unpeeled Granny Smith apple, cored
    and cut into chunks

1 pkg (12 oz) fresh or thawed frozen
    cranberries

⅓ c honey

Orange zest strips

1. Process orange in food processor until finely chopped (in batches if necessary). Add dates and apple and coarsely chop. Add cranberries and coarsely chop.

2. Transfer to medium bowl and fold in honey. Store in airtight container and refrigerate. Garnish with orange zest.

Makes 8 servings

Per serving: 105 cal, 1 g pro, 28 g carb, 0 g fat, 0 g sat fat, 0 mg chol, 3 g fiber, 2 mg sodium

Diet Exchanges: 0 milk, 0 vegetable, 1 fruit, 1 starch/bread, 0 meat, 0 fat

CHICKEN AND TURKEY MAIN DISHES

Soft Tacos with Chicken and Kidney Beans

Photo on page 285

1 whole boneless, skinless chicken breast (1 lb), trimmed and sliced thin

1 clove garlic, minced

Pinch of ground red pepper

3 Tbsp canola oil, divided

1 c chopped onion

$1/3$ c sodium-free canned diced tomatoes

2 c rinsed and drained canned red kidney beans

8 low-fat whole wheat tortillas (8" diameter)

$1/2$ c cubed avocado

1 c salsa (optional)

$1/2$ c low-fat sour cream (optional)

1. In small bowl, combine chicken with garlic, red pepper, and 2 tablespoons of the oil. Season with salt and freshly ground black pepper. Toss well to coat chicken.

2. In medium nonstick skillet over medium-high heat, cook chicken 7 to 10 minutes, turning frequently, until no longer pink and juices run clear. Transfer chicken to plate.

3. In same skillet over medium heat, sauté onion in remaining 1 tablespoon oil about 3 minutes or until translucent. Stir in tomatoes (with juice). Stir in beans, reduce heat to low, and cook until heated through.

4. Warm tortillas in microwave or toaster oven. Fill each tortilla with bean mixture, chicken, and 1 tablespoon of the avocado. Serve with salsa and sour cream, if desired.

Makes 4 servings

Per serving: 580 cal, 47 g pro, 56 g carb, 19 g fat, 1.5 g sat fat, 65 mg chol, 18 g fiber, 445 mg sodium

Diet Exchanges: 0 milk, 1 vegetable, 0 fruit, 2 starch/bread, 4 meat, 2.5 fat

Grape-Ful Chicken

1 sm butternut squash, cut into 1" cubes
   (about 2$\frac{1}{2}$ c)

1 c pearl onions

4 skinless, bone-in chicken breast halves
   (1$\frac{1}{4}$ lb)

$\frac{1}{4}$ c chopped fresh tarragon

2 tsp olive oil

1$\frac{1}{2}$ c chicken broth

1 Tbsp cornstarch

2 c seedless red grapes

1. Place squash cubes on microwaveable plate and sprinkle with water. Microwave on high 4 minutes.

2. Drop onions in boiling water. Cook 3 minutes. Drain, then immerse onions in cold water. Cut root end of each onion and squeeze gently to remove outer skin.

3. Sprinkle both sides of chicken breasts with salt and pepper and rub with tarragon.

4. Heat oil in large Dutch oven over medium-high heat. Add chicken and sauté 3 minutes per side, until thermometer inserted in thickest portion registers 170°F and juices run clear.

Add squash, onions, and 1 cup of the broth, and bring to a simmer. Reduce heat to medium, cover, and cook 15 minutes.

5. Using a slotted spoon, remove chicken and vegetables from pot and transfer to serving platter, reserving liquid in pot.

6. Dissolve cornstarch in remaining $\frac{1}{2}$ cup broth. Add mixture to remaining liquid in pot, add grapes, and simmer 1 minute or until liquid thickens. Pour sauce over chicken and vegetables, and serve immediately.

Makes 4 servings

Per serving: 360 cal, 36 g pro, 41 g carb, 6 g fat, 2 g sat fat, 85 mg chol, 6 g fiber, 480 mg sodium

Diet Exchanges: 0 milk, 1 vegetable, 1 fruit, 0 starch/bread, 5 meat, 1 fat

One-Skillet Chicken

1/4 c all-purpose flour

1/4 tsp salt

1/4 tsp black pepper

1 lb boneless, skinless chicken breast
    cutlets (about 1/4" thick)

4 tsp olive oil

1 can (14 1/2 oz) diced tomatoes primavera
    (with zucchini, bell peppers, and
    carrots)

1. In shallow bowl, combine flour, salt,
and pepper.

2. Coat chicken with seasoned flour.
Tap off excess.

3. In large nonstick skillet, heat 2
teaspoons of the oil over medium-high
heat. Brown half of the cutlets 3 minutes per side or until no longer pink
and juices run clear. Remove to large
plate and cover with foil to keep warm.
Repeat with remaining oil and cutlets.

4. Add tomatoes (with juice) to skillet
and simmer 2 minutes or until heated
through.

5. Divide cutlets equally among 4 plates
and spoon an equal portion of sauce
over top.

Makes 4 servings

Per serving: 230 cal, 28 g pro, 13 g carb, 6 g fat,
1 g sat fat, 66 mg chol, 2 g fiber, 610 mg sodium

Diet Exchanges: 0 milk, 1.5 vegetable, 0 fruit,
0.5 starch/bread, 4 meat, 1 fat

Chicken Stir-Fry

2 tsp reduced-sodium soy sauce

1 tsp honey

2 tsp sesame oil

1 lg bunch asparagus (about 1 3/4 lb),
    trimmed and cut on diagonal into
    1" pieces

1 clove garlic, minced, or 1 tsp bottled
    minced garlic

2 1/2 c sliced cooked chicken breast

1. Combine soy sauce and honey in
small bowl. Set aside.

2. Heat oil in large skillet or wok over
medium-high heat. Add asparagus and
garlic. Cook 4 minutes, stirring frequently.

3. Toss in chicken and soy sauce–honey
mixture. Heat thoroughly, remove from
pan with tongs.

Makes 4 servings

Per serving: 200 cal, 30 g pro, 7 g carb, 5 g fat,
1 g sat fat, 75 mg chol, 2 g fiber, 210 mg sodium

Diet Exchanges: 0 milk, 1 vegetable, 0 fruit,
0 starch/bread, 4 meat, 1 fat

Pesto Chicken

$^1/_2$ c seasoned dried bread crumbs

2 Tbsp finely chopped, drained sun-dried
  tomatoes packed in oil, 1 Tbsp oil set
  aside

$^1/_2$ tsp cracked black pepper

$^1/_4$ c prepared pesto

4 bone-in, skinless chicken breast halves

1. Preheat oven to 375°F. Coat 13" × 9"
baking pan with cooking spray.

2. In shallow bowl, combine bread
crumbs, tomatoes, and pepper. Spread
pesto on top of chicken breasts, then
dip in crumb mixture, pressing to coat
evenly. Arrange chicken, breast sides
up, in pan. Drizzle with reserved
tomato oil.

3. Bake 40 minutes or until thermometer inserted in thickest portion registers
170°F and juices run clear.

Makes 4 servings

Per serving: 300 cal, 31 g pro, 12 g carb, 13 g fat,
2.5 g sat fat, 70 mg chol, 1 g fiber, 610 mg sodium

Diet Exchanges: 0 milk, 0 vegetable, 0 fruit,
1 bread, 4 meat, 2 fat

Jamaican Grilled Chicken

$^1/_4$ c jarred chutney

1 tsp Caribbean-style hot-pepper sauce (we
  used Pickapeppa)

4 boneless, skinless chicken breasts (about
  6 oz each)

2 Tbsp Jamaican jerk seasoning

1 lb fresh asparagus, trimmed

1. Preheat grill to medium-high. In
small bowl, mix chutney and hot-
pepper sauce and set aside. Rub
chicken with jerk seasoning.

2. Grill breasts about 6 minutes per
side, brushing every few minutes with
chutney mixture, until thermometer
inserted in thickest portion registers
160°F and juices run clear.

3. Meanwhile, grill asparagus about
6 minutes, turning occasionally.
Remove chicken and asparagus from
grill and arrange on platter to serve.

Makes 4 servings

Per serving: 242 cal, 42 g pro, 11 g carb, 2 g fat,
0.5 g sat fat, 99 mg chol, 3 g fiber, 567 mg sodium

Diet Exchanges: 0 milk, 2 vegetable, 0 fruit,
0 starch/bread, 5.5 meat, 0 fat

Oregano Chicken

6 sm boneless, skinless chicken breast
    halves (2¹⁄₄ lb total)

1 c coarsely chopped fresh oregano leaves

4 scallions, trimmed and thinly sliced

¹⁄₂ c balsamic vinegar

¹⁄₄ c extra-virgin olive oil

2 tsp freshly cracked black pepper

³⁄₄ tsp salt

1. Place chicken breast halves between 2 sheets of plastic wrap. Using mallet or heavy pan, pound meat until it is ³⁄₄" thick.

2. Place chicken in shallow dish. In small bowl, whisk oregano, scallions, vinegar, oil, pepper, and salt. Pour mixture over chicken and flip to coat both sides. Cover and chill about 2 hours, turning once.

3. Heat grill to medium for indirect heat. (If using charcoal grill, position coals on one half of grill. If using gas grill, heat one side to high, the other to low.) Wipe grill grates with vegetable oil.

4. Remove chicken from marinade, reserving marinade. Place chicken on hottest section of grill. Cook 6 minutes, turning once. Move chicken to cooler section of grill and cook 6 minutes, turning once, until thermometer inserted in thickest portion registers 160°F and juices run clear.

5. Pour marinade into small saucepan and place on hottest part of grill. Bring to a boil for 5 minutes.

6. Arrange chicken breasts on plates and drizzle with warm marinade.

Makes 6 servings

Per serving: 291 cal, 40 g pro, 5 g carb, 12 g fat, 2 g sat fat, 99 mg chol, 1 g fiber, 410 mg sodium

Diet Exchanges: 0 milk, 0.5 vegetable, 0 fruit, 0 starch/bread, 5.5 meat, 2 fat

Tandoori Chicken

1 sm onion, quartered

¹⁄₂ c low-fat plain Greek-style yogurt

5 cloves garlic

¹⁄₂" piece ginger, peeled

³⁄₄ tsp ground coriander

³⁄₄ tsp ground cumin

¹⁄₂ tsp ground allspice

¹⁄₂ tsp ground cinnamon

¹⁄₂ tsp ground turmeric

¹⁄₄ tsp freshly ground black pepper

¹⁄₄ tsp ground red pepper

8 skinless, bone-in chicken thighs (about 3 lb)

$^1/_2$ tsp salt

1. Combine onion, yogurt, garlic, ginger, coriander, cumin, allspice, cinnamon, turmeric, black pepper, and red pepper in food processor and blend until smooth.

2. Prick chicken all over with sharp knife and place in shallow dish. Add marinade, turning to coat chicken completely. Cover and chill overnight or up to 24 hours.

3. Coat grill rack with cooking spray and preheat grill to high.

4. Remove chicken from marinade (discard marinade). Season chicken with salt and grill 12 minutes, turning once. Reduce heat to medium and grill 12 to 15 minutes longer, flipping once, until thermometer inserted in thickest portion reads 170°F and thighs are no longer pink inside.

Makes 4 servings

Per serving: 200 cal, 30 g pro, 5 g carb, 6 g fat, 2 g sat fat, 116 mg chol, 1 g fiber, 420 mg sodium

Diet Exchanges: 0 milk, 0.5 vegetable, 0 fruit, 0 starch/bread, 4 meat, 1 fat

Santa Fe Pizza

1 prebaked pizza crust (12")

$^1/_2$ c guacamole

1 pkg (10 oz) sliced cooked, Southwest-style chicken breast

$^1/_2$ c roasted red peppers, drained and sliced

2 c shredded pepper Jack cheese (8 oz)

1. Preheat oven to 350°F. Place pizza crust on oiled baking sheet.

2. Spread guacamole evenly over crust. Top with chicken and peppers and sprinkle with cheese.

3. Bake pizza 15 minutes or until cheese bubbles and slightly browns. Cut pizza into wedges.

Makes 4 servings

Per serving: 590 cal, 34 g pro, 49 g carb, 30 g fat, 12 g sat fat, 85 mg chol, 4 g fiber, 1,440 mg sodium

Diet Exchanges: 0 milk, 0 vegetable, 0 fruit, 3 starch/bread, 3$^1/_2$ meat, 4 fat

Chicken Potpie with Sweet Potato Biscuits

Biscuits

3/4 c all-purpose flour

1/4 c whole wheat flour

1 1/2 tsp baking powder

1/4 tsp salt

2 Tbsp unsalted butter, cold

1/3 c 1% milk

1/4 c mashed sweet potato

Filling

2 Tbsp unsalted butter

1 c chopped onion (1/2" pieces)

1/4 c chopped celery (1/2" pieces)

1 c chopped potatoes (1/2" pieces)

1/2 c chopped carrots (1/2" pieces)

3/4 lb boneless, skinless chicken breast, cut into 3/4" pieces

1 Tbsp all-purpose flour

1 c 1% milk

1 c reduced-sodium chicken broth

1 bay leaf

2 tsp chopped parsley

1 1/2 tsp chopped fresh tarragon

1. Preheat oven to 450°F.

2. To prepare biscuits: In medium bowl, combine flours, baking powder, and salt and mix well. Cut butter into small pieces and add to flour mixture. Using fingertips, work butter into flour until it has consistency of cornmeal.

3. In small bowl, combine milk and sweet potato and mix well with fork. Add to flour mixture and stir quickly just until it forms a ball. Turn dough onto lightly floured surface and knead 14 times. Do not overwork or dough will become tough.

4. Pat dough out until it is 1/2" thick. Cut into rounds with biscuit cutter. Gather scraps, pat out, and cut again until all dough is used. Place on cookie sheet and bake 8 to 10 minutes or until bottoms of biscuits are golden brown.

5. To prepare filling: Melt butter in medium saucepan over medium heat. Add onion and celery and cook about 2 minutes or until onion is translucent. Add potatoes and carrots and cook about 10 minutes or until hard vegetables soften. Add chicken and cook 3 minutes. Stir in flour and cook 3 minutes longer. Add milk, broth, and bay leaf and cook about 8 minutes or until vegetables are tender.

6. Stir in parsley and tarragon, season with salt and pepper, and cook 5 minutes or until chicken is fully cooked. Remove and discard bay leaf.

7. To serve, place a bottom half of biscuit in each of 4 bowls, add potpie filling, and cap with biscuit tops.

Makes 4 servings

Per serving: 497 cal, 30 g pro, 60 g carb, 14 g fat, 8 g sat fat, 83 mg chol, 5 g fiber, 561 mg sodium

Diet Exchanges: 0.5 milk, 1 vegetable, 0 fruit, 2 starch/bread, 3 meat, 2 fat

Ginger-Sesame Stir-Fry

1 c sushi rice, rinsed and drained

$1^1/_4$ c water

2 Tbsp canola oil

1 Tbsp grated fresh ginger

4 cloves garlic, minced

4 scallions, thinly sliced

1 lb boneless, skinless chicken breasts, thinly sliced

$1^1/_2$ bunches broccolini (1 lb), sliced diagonally, or $3^1/_2$ c broccoli florets

1 red bell pepper, cored and thinly sliced

2 tsp cornstarch, dissolved in $^2/_3$ c water

$^1/_2$ tsp salt

2 tsp toasted sesame oil

1. Combine rice and water in small saucepan and bring to a boil. Reduce heat to low, cover, and simmer 20 minutes. Remove from heat and let stand 10 minutes without lifting cover.

2. Preheat wok or large heavy-bottomed skillet over high heat 30 seconds. Add canola oil, ginger, garlic, and scallions and stir 1 minute, until scallions begin to soften. Add chicken and continue to stir 2 minutes, until surfaces of chicken are mostly white.

3. Add broccolini or broccoli and pepper and stir 1 minute or until slightly softened. Add cornstarch mixture and salt, stirring to coat ingredients. Bring to a boil, reduce heat to medium, and allow liquid to reduce to a thick sauce, about 1 minute. Drizzle with sesame oil.

4. Wet hands and shape rice into 4 balls. Serve with stir-fry.

Makes 4 servings

Per serving: 450 cal, 34 g pro, 51 g carb, 11 g fat, 1.5 g sat fat, 66 mg chol, 4 g fiber, 406 mg sodium

Diet Exchanges: 0 milk, 2 vegetable, 0 fruit, 2 starch/bread, 4 meat, 2 fat

Grilled Ginger-Soy Chicken

¼ c reduced-sodium soy sauce

2 Tbsp minced fresh ginger

2 Tbsp honey

2 Tbsp miso paste

1 Tbsp minced garlic

2 tsp toasted sesame oil

¼ tsp red-pepper flakes

8 boneless, skinless chicken breast halves
    (3–4 lb)

½ tsp kosher salt

1. Combine soy sauce, ginger, honey, miso, garlic, oil, and red-pepper flakes in shallow baking dish or large resealable plastic bag. Add chicken, turn to coat, cover, and chill at least 2 hours.

2. Heat grill to medium for indirect heat. If using charcoal grill, position coals on one-half of grill. If using gas grill, heat one side to high, the other to low. Lightly oil grill grates.

3. Remove chicken from marinade. Discard marinade. Season chicken with salt.

4. Grill chicken 10 minutes over hottest section of grill, turning once. Move to cooler section of grill and cook 10 minutes longer or until thermometer inserted in thickest portion registers 160°F and juices run clear.

Makes 8 servings

Per serving: 210 cal, 40 g pro, 4 g carb, 3 g fat, 0.5 g sat fat, 99 mg chol, 0 g fiber, 423 mg sodium

Diet Exchanges: 0 milk, 0 vegetable, 0 fruit, 0 starch/bread, 5.5 meat, 0 fat

Soba Noodles with Chicken and Snow Peas

8 oz dry soba noodles or whole wheat
    spaghetti

2 Tbsp honey

2 Tbsp freshly squeezed lime juice

2 Tbsp rice-wine vinegar

2 Tbsp reduced-sodium soy sauce

1 Tbsp grated fresh ginger

¼ tsp red-pepper flakes

2 Tbsp peanut oil

2 c julienned fresh snow peas

2 red bell peppers, cored and thinly sliced
    lengthwise

2 c shredded Grilled Ginger-Soy Chicken
    (see recipe on the left)

1 c grated carrots

¼ c coarsely chopped fresh cilantro

1. Cook noodles per package directions. Rinse with cold water, drain, and set aside.

2. Whisk together honey, lime juice, vinegar, soy sauce, ginger, and red-pepper flakes in large bowl. Whisk in oil in steady stream.

3. Add noodles, snow peas, peppers, chicken, carrots, and cilantro to bowl and toss well. Season with salt to taste.

Makes 6 servings

Per serving: 292 cal, 19 g pro, 45 g carb, 5.5 g fat, 1 g sat fat, 26 mg chol, 4 g fiber, 388 mg sodium

Diet Exchanges: 0 milk, 1 vegetable, 0 fruit, 2 starch/bread, 1.5 meat, 1 fat

Linguine Primavera Parmesan with Chicken

8 oz fresh linguine

4 Tbsp olive oil

4 c cut-up mixed vegetables such as broccoli, carrots, bell peppers, and zucchini

2 pkg (6 oz) grilled chicken breast strips

²/₃ c grated Parmesan cheese

1. Half-fill large saucepan with salted water and bring to a boil. Add linguine and cook 2 minutes, then drain and keep hot.

2. Heat oil in large nonstick skillet over medium-high heat. Sauté vegetables 5 minutes or until crisp-tender. Add chicken and pasta. Cook and toss mixture 2 minutes or until heated through. Add Parmesan and toss well.

Makes 4 servings

Per serving: 470 cal, 26 g pro, 44 g carb, 22 g fat, 5 g sat fat, 90 mg chol, 5 g fiber, 640 mg sodium

Diet Exchanges: 0 milk, 1 vegetable, 0 fruit, 2.5 starch/bread, 2 meat, 3.5 fat

Summer Rolls with Peanut Dipping Sauce

Sauce

$^1/_2$ c fat-free reduced-sodium chicken broth

$^1/_3$ c peanut butter

2 Tbsp reduced-sodium soy sauce

1 Tbsp freshly squeezed lime juice

1 Tbsp rice-wine vinegar

1–2 tsp chile paste

Rolls

2 oz dry rice vermicelli (thin Asian rice-flour noodles)

8 round (8"–9"diameter) rice-paper sheets (aka spring-roll wrappers) or lg lettuce leaves

$^1/_2$ c basil leaves

1 c julienned cucumber, with peel

1 c julienned carrots

1 c thinly sliced Grilled Ginger-Soy Chicken (see page 320)

$^1/_2$ c mint leaves

1. Combine sauce ingredients in small saucepan over medium-low heat. Cook, whisking until smooth, 2 to 3 minutes. Remove from heat and set aside.

2. Cook rice vermicelli per package directions (cooked yield should be about 1 cup). Rinse with cold water and drain.

3. Soak 1 rice-paper sheet in warm water 30 to 90 seconds or until soft. Carefully transfer to clean towel and blot dry. Place 3 or 4 basil leaves along bottom third of sheet (leaving $^1/_2$" margin along edges). Layer $^1/_8$ cup of the rice vermicelli on top of basil, followed by $^1/_8$ of the cucumber, carrots, chicken, and mint leaves. Starting from the bottom, roll rice paper around the filling. Fold sides up and continue rolling until roll is sealed completely. Repeat with remaining sheets and filling. Cut each roll in half crosswise and serve with peanut sauce.

Makes 8 servings

Per serving: 134 cal, 8 g pro, 11 g carb, 7 g fat, 1 g sat fat, 10 mg chol, 2 g fiber, 254 mg sodium

Diet Exchanges: 0 milk, 0.5 vegetable, 0 fruit, 1 starch/bread, 1 meat, 1 fat

Oven-Fried Chicken

$^2/_3$ c buttermilk or fat-free plain yogurt

2 Tbsp lime juice

$^1/_2$ tsp salt

$^1/_2$ tsp freshly ground black pepper

$1^1/_4$ c yellow cornmeal

6 split chicken breasts, skin and visible fat removed

1. Preheat oven to 425°F. Coat large baking sheet with sides with cooking spray.

2. In large bowl, combine buttermilk or yogurt, lime juice, salt, and pepper. Place cornmeal in pie plate.

3. Dip chicken in buttermilk mixture, turning to coat well. (Chicken may be marinated in buttermilk mixture in refrigerator up to 1 day.)

4. One at a time, roll chicken pieces in cornmeal, pressing to coat thoroughly. Place chicken, skinned side up, on baking sheet. Discard any remaining buttermilk mixture and cornmeal.

5. Coat chicken well with cooking spray. Bake 40 minutes or until thermometer inserted in thickest portion registers 170°F and juices run clear.

Makes 6 servings

Per serving: 230 cal, 23 g pro, 29 g carb, 1.5 g fat, 0 g sat fat, 50 mg chol, 1 g fiber, 280 mg sodium

Diet Exchanges: 0 milk, 1 vegetable, 0 fruit, 1½ starch/bread, 3 meat, 0 fat

Turkey Tostada

4 whole wheat flour tortillas (6" diameter)

1 c shredded cooked turkey

½ c prepared black bean and corn salsa (we used Desert Pepper Trading Company)

½ c reduced-fat mozzarella cheese

6 Tbsp low-fat plain yogurt

2 Tbsp chopped cilantro

1. Preheat oven to 350°F. Place tortillas on baking sheet and heat 7 minutes or until crisp. Set aside.

2. Combine turkey and salsa in small microwaveable bowl. Microwave on high until warmed through, about 3 minutes. Divide turkey-salsa mixture among tortillas and sprinkle each with 2 tablespoons of cheese. Top each tostada with 1½ tablespoons of yogurt and ½ tablespoon of cilantro.

Makes 4 servings

Per serving: 270 cal, 20 g pro, 28 g carb, 7 g fat, 2.5 g sat fat, 35 mg chol, 2 g fiber, 530 mg sodium

Diet Exchanges: 0 milk, 0 vegetable, 0 fruit, 1.5 starch/bread, 2 meat, 1 fat

Roast Turkey with Apple and Orange Pan Juices

Photo on page 286

1 (12–14 lb) turkey, fresh or thawed

1 tsp salt (optional)

$\frac{1}{4}$ tsp freshly ground black pepper

1 rib celery, with leaves, chopped

1 unpeeled Golden Delicious apple, cut
    into 8 wedges

1 unpeeled navel orange, cut into
    8 wedges

1 onion, cut into 8 wedges

$\frac{1}{2}$ c snipped sprigs thyme

4 Tbsp olive oil

$4\frac{1}{2}$ c fat-free chicken broth

2 c unsweetened apple juice

1 Tbsp all-purpose flour

1. Remove turkey from refrigerator 1 hour before roasting. Place in sink. Remove wrapping and reach inside cavity to remove bag of giblets. Discard or reserve for other use. Rinse turkey inside and out with cold running water. Use paper towels to dry inside and out. If not using a nonstick roasting rack, lightly coat rack with cooking spray. Place turkey breast-side up on roasting rack set in large roasting pan.

2. Move oven rack to lowest position. Preheat oven to 425°F.

3. Season turkey inside with salt, if using, and pepper. In large bowl, combine celery, apple, orange, onion, and thyme. Stuff large cavity with three-quarters mixture. Pull skin over opening and secure with wooden picks or small metal skewers. Stuff neck cavity with remaining mixture. Secure flap as above. Using cotton kitchen string, tie drumsticks together and tuck wing tips under body.

4. Rub turkey with 2 tablespoons of the oil. Cut doubled cheesecloth large enough to cover surface of turkey. In medium bowl, drizzle cheesecloth with remaining 2 tablespoons oil. Squeeze to distribute evenly. Cover surface of bird with cheesecloth.

5. Add 4 cups of the broth to pan. Roast bird 30 minutes. Reduce oven temperature to 325°F. Roast $2\frac{1}{2}$ to 3 hours longer, basting bird with pan juices every 30 minutes. Remove from oven when meat thermometer inserted in meaty part of thigh (but not touching bone) registers 165°F. Transfer to cutting board. Remove cheesecloth.

Tent bird with large piece of foil and let stand 30 to 45 minutes. (Temperature will increase to 170°F while bird stands.)

6. While turkey stands, pour drippings into fat-separator measuring cup or 4-cup liquid measure and let stand 10 minutes. Spoon off and discard fat that rises.

7. Prepare light gravy: Add apple juice to drippings; there should be about 6 cups total. If there's less, add broth to equal 6 cups. Pour into medium saucepan and bring to a boil over medium-high heat. Stirring occasionally, boil until reduced by half. In small bowl, blend flour with $1/4$ cup of broth (can also use water or apple juice). Whisk in ladleful of hot broth and then another. Whisk into saucepan and heat, stirring, to boil. Gravy should be slightly thickened without any visible lumps (strain if lumpy). Add salt and pepper to taste. Keep warm until ready to serve, then transfer to serving bowl or gravy boat. Makes 3 to $3 1/2$ cups gravy, or about twelve $1/4$-cup servings.

8. Remove filling from turkey and discard. Carve turkey and arrange on serving platter. Garnish with seasonal greenery, such as crab apples, or fresh fruits and herbs.

Makes 12 servings

Turkey, with skin, per serving (10 ounces): 470 cal, 58 g pro, 0 g carb, 25 g fat, 6 g sat fat, 180 mg chol, 0 g fiber, 190 mg sodium

Diet Exchanges: 0 milk, 0 vegetable, 0 fruit, 0 starch/bread, 8.5 meat, 3.5 fat

Turkey, without skin, per serving (10 ounces): 350 cal, 58 g pro, 0 g carb, 11 g fat, 2.5 g sat fat, 165 mg chol, 0 g fiber, 190 mg sodium

Diet Exchanges: 0 milk, 0 vegetable, 0 fruit, 0 starch/bread, 8.5 meat, 1 fat

Gravy per serving ($1/4$ cup): 45 cal, 2 g pro, 5 g carb, 2 g fat, 0.5 g sat fat, 0 mg chol, 0 g fiber, 130 mg sodium

Diet Exchanges: 0 milk, 0 vegetable, 0 fruit, 0.5 starch/bread, 0 meat, 0.5 fat

Easy Turkey Chili

1 lb lean ground turkey

1 can (14 oz) Mexican-style diced tomatoes

1 can (15$\frac{1}{2}$ oz) black beans, rinsed and
    drained

1 can (14 oz) whole-kernel sweet corn,
    drained

1 pkg (1$\frac{1}{4}$ oz) dry chili mix

$\frac{1}{4}$ c water

1. In large nonstick skillet, brown turkey over medium-high heat until no longer pink.

2. Add tomatoes (with juice), beans, corn, chili mix, and water. Cook over low heat 10 minutes, stirring occasionally.

Makes 4 servings

Per serving: 320 cal, 27 g pro, 31 g carb, 11 g fat, 2.5 g sat fat, 90 mg chol, 8 g fiber, 1,230 mg sodium

Diet Exchanges: 0 milk, 1 vegetable, 0 fruit, 1$\frac{1}{2}$ starch/bread, 3 meat, 0 fat

BEEF AND PORK MAIN DISHES

Mustard-Crusted London Broil

Photo on page 351

$\frac{3}{4}$ c panko

1 Tbsp fresh thyme leaves, chopped

1 lb top-round London broil, trimmed

1$\frac{1}{2}$ Tbsp Dijon mustard

2 cloves garlic, minced

1. Arrange oven rack on top position. Preheat oven to 450°F. Fit baking or roasting pan with wire rack.

2. Mix panko and thyme on a plate.

3. Season both sides of London broil with salt and pepper to taste. Combine mustard and garlic in small bowl and cover meat with mixture.

4. Coat London broil with panko mixture, pressing crumbs into meat so they stick. Discard remaining crumbs. Place meat on rack and coat top and sides thoroughly with olive oil spray.

5. Roast 16 to 18 minutes for medium doneness or until crumbs are golden and desired doneness is reached. If crumbs begin browning too much, cover beef loosely with foil. Remove from oven and let stand 10 minutes. Slice into thin strips and serve.

Makes 4 servings

Per serving: 230 cal, 28 g pro, 9 g carb, 8.5 g fat, 3 g sat fat, 50 mg chol, 0 g fiber, 230 mg sodium

Diet Exchanges: 0 milk, 0 vegetable, 0 fruit, 0.5 starch/bread, 3.5 meat, 1 fat

Korean Barbecued Beef

5 scallions, finely chopped

5 cloves garlic, minced

2 tsp sesame seeds, toasted

3 Tbsp reduced-sodium soy sauce

2 Tbsp sugar

1 Tbsp water

2 tsp toasted sesame oil

1 tsp rice-wine vinegar

1 lb beef tenderloin, trimmed and sliced into
　　$1/4$" thick medallions

1. Grind scallions, garlic, and sesame seeds in small food processor or with mortar and pestle. Stir in soy sauce, sugar, water, oil, and vinegar.

2. Pour into shallow dish. Add beef, turning slices to coat. Cover and chill 45 minutes.

3. Preheat grill to high for direct heat.

4. Remove beef from marinade (discard marinade). Grill 2 to 3 minutes, turning once.

Makes 4 servings

Per serving: 244 cal, 27 g pro, 10 g carb, 10.5 g fat, 3 g sat fat, 76 mg chol, 1 g fiber, 521 mg sodium

Diet Exchanges: 0 milk, 0 vegetable, 0 fruit, 0.5 starch/bread, 4 meat, 1.5 fat

Spiced Kofta Sliders

$^1/_3$ c med bulgur

$^1/_3$ lb ground lamb

$^1/_3$ lb 95% lean ground beef

$^1/_2$ med onion, grated

4 cloves garlic, minced

$^1/_4$ c finely chopped mint

$1^1/_2$ tsp red curry paste

$^3/_4$ tsp ground cumin

$^1/_2$ tsp ground allspice

$^1/_4$ tsp ground coriander

$^1/_2$ med cucumber, grated and spun dry in salad spinner (about $^1/_2$ c)

$^1/_3$ c low-fat plain Greek-style yogurt

$^1/_4$ tsp freshly ground black pepper

12 lg lettuce leaves

1 med tomato, chopped (about $^1/_2$ c)

1. Soak bulgur in $^1/_3$ cup hot water 1 hour.

2. Combine bulgur and lamb, beef, onion, garlic, mint, curry paste, cumin, allspice, and coriander. Chill, covered, 30 minutes.

3. Mix cucumber, yogurt, and pepper in small bowl. Season with salt.

4. Preheat grill to medium-high. Shape meat mixture into 12 balls and flatten into thick miniburgers. Season with salt.

5. Grill patties 4 to 8 minutes, turning once, until thermometer inserted in center registers 160°F. Wrap each patty in a lettuce leaf and serve with yogurt sauce and tomato.

Makes 4 servings

Per serving: 247 cal, 19 g pro, 17 g carb, 12 g fat, 5 g sat fat, 52 mg chol, 4 g fiber, 574 mg sodium

Diet Exchanges: 0 milk, 1 vegetable, 0 fruit, 0.5 starch/bread, 2 meat, 1.5 fat

Moroccan Meatballs in Tomato Sauce

1¼ lb ground beef or lamb

1 Tbsp paprika, divided

2 tsp ground cumin

Leaves from 12 lg parsley sprigs, chopped

1 lg clove garlic

1 can (15 oz) diced tomatoes, drained

¼ c olive oil

3 Tbsp tomato paste

1 sm onion, cut into chunks

8 oz spaghetti

1. Place ground beef or lamb in large bowl. Add 1½ teaspoons of the paprika, 1 teaspoon of the cumin, and half of the parsley. Mix or knead to thoroughly distribute flavorings through meat. Roll into 1" balls and place on plate. Bring large pot of water to a boil for pasta.

2. In food processor, combine garlic, tomatoes, oil, tomato paste, and onion. Process until mixed. Add remaining paprika, cumin, and parsley. Process until nearly smooth. Scrape into medium pot or deep 10" skillet. Place over medium heat, bring to boil, and cook 2 to 3 minutes.

3. Remove pan from heat. Nestle meatballs into sauce in one layer. Swirl pan gently to cover meatballs with sauce. Place over medium heat, positioning lid slightly ajar, and cook 10 to 12 minutes, until meatballs are cooked through and no longer pink. While meatballs are cooking, add spaghetti to boiling water and prepare per package directions. Drain and place spaghetti in a large serving dish. Serve meatballs and sauce over spaghetti.

Makes 4 servings

Per serving: 541 cal, 37 g pro, 51 g carb, 21 g fat, 4.6 g sat fat, 75 mg chol, 4 g fiber, 317 mg sodium

Diet Exchanges: 0 milk, 1.5 vegetable, 0 fruit, 3 starch/bread, 4 meat, 3 fat

Hearty Brussels Sprouts with Sausage

1 lb low-fat Italian chicken sausages (garlic or mild)

2 tsp olive oil

$1/4$ c slivered almonds

6 cardamom pods, cracked

$1/4$ tsp ground cloves

$1/4$ tsp cumin seed

$1/8$ tsp white pepper

$1^1/2$ lb Brussels sprouts, quartered

$1/2$ c reduced-sodium chicken broth

1. Remove sausage casings and discard. Crumble sausage meat with a fork.

2. Warm oil in 12" skillet over high heat. Add sausage, almonds, cardamom, cloves, cumin, and pepper. Cook, stirring, until sausage is no longer pink and almonds become golden in places, about 6 minutes.

3. Add Brussels sprouts and broth. Stir to combine. Cover tightly and cook 15 minutes or until sprouts can be easily pierced with fork. Uncover and continue cooking until most of liquid in pan has evaporated, about 3 minutes. Serve.

Makes 4 servings

Per serving: 290 cal, 31 g pro, 17 g carb, 13 g fat, 2.5 g sat fat, 35 mg chol, 7 g fiber, 53 mg sodium

Diet Exchanges: 0 milk, 3 vegetable, 0 fruit, 0 starch/bread, 0.5 meat, 1 fat

Herbed Pork Roast

Photo on page 352

1 lb pork tenderloin (1 lg or 2 sm), trimmed

1 tsp olive oil

$1/8$ tsp ground red pepper

$1/8$ tsp garlic powder

$1/8$ tsp salt

$1/8$ tsp black pepper

$1/4$ c chopped flat-leaf parsley leaves

2 Tbsp chopped fresh rosemary leaves

1. Preheat oven to 450°F.

2. Rub pork with oil and sprinkle evenly with red pepper, garlic powder, salt, and black pepper.

3. Press parsley and rosemary evenly over roast so they stick. Transfer pork to small nonstick baking or roasting pan. Tuck tapered end of tenderloin under itself for even cooking. Roast 18 to 22 minutes or until thermometer inserted in center reaches 155°F and juices run clear. Let stand 10 minutes before slicing.

Makes 4 servings

Per serving: 150 cal, 24 g pro, 1 g carb, 5 g fat, 1.5 g sat fat, 75 mg chol, 0 g fiber, 130 mg sodium

Diet Exchanges: 0 milk, 0 vegetable, 0 fruit, 0 starch/bread, 3.5 meat, 0.5 fat

Pork Chops with Cabbage

4 center-cut pork chops (4 oz each), trimmed

4 tsp Dijon mustard

$\frac{1}{2}$ head red cabbage (about 16 oz), cored and thinly sliced

2 Granny Smith apples, peeled and grated + additional slices

$\frac{1}{4}$ tsp salt

1 tsp + 1 Tbsp canola oil

1 Tbsp grated fresh ginger

$\frac{1}{2}$ tsp ground cinnamon

$\frac{1}{4}$ tsp ground cloves

1 Tbsp pure maple syrup

2 tsp cider vinegar

1. Brush both sides of pork chops with mustard and set aside. Toss cabbage, grated apples, and salt in large bowl.

2. In large skillet with lid, warm 1 teaspoon of the oil over medium-low heat. Add ginger, cinnamon, and cloves. Stir 10 to 15 seconds until fragrant. Add cabbage-apple mixture and maple syrup. Stir, reduce heat to low, cover, and cook until ingredients are soft and cooked through, about 30 minutes.

3. Meanwhile, heat remaining 1 tablespoon oil in heavy skillet over medium-high heat. Arrange pork in single layer. Cook, flipping halfway through, about 9 minutes or until thermometer inserted in center of a chop reaches 160°F and juices run clear.

4. Remove cover from cabbage, stir in vinegar, and raise heat to medium. Cook until liquid mostly evaporates, 5 minutes. Serve each chop with a mound of cabbage. Garnish with apple slices, if desired.

Makes 4 servings

Per serving: 280 cal, 27 g pro, 20 g carb, 11 g fat, 2.5 g sat fat, 70 mg chol, 4 g fiber, 368 mg sodium

Diet Exchanges: 0 milk, 1 vegetable, 0.5 fruit, 0 starch/bread, 3.5 meat, 2 fat

Roasted Dijon Pork with Baked Apples

4 thinly sliced, center-cut, boneless pork
    loin chops (4–5 oz each)

2 Tbsp Dijon mustard

$^1/_2$ c unsweetened applesauce

16 Golden Delicious apple slices ($^1/_4$" thick)

1. Preheat oven to 375°F.

2. Place pork chops in large baking dish. Spread top of each with mustard, then applesauce.

3. Coat apple slices with butter-flavored cooking spray, then place 4 slices on top of each chop. Bake 20 minutes or until thermometer inserted in center of a chop registers 160°F and juices run clear. Season with salt and pepper, if desired, before serving.

Makes 4 servings

Per serving: 230 cal, 22 g pro, 11 g carb, 12 g fat, 4 g sat fat, 60 mg chol, 2 g fiber, 590 mg sodium

Diet Exchanges: 0 milk, 1 fruit, 0 vegetable, 0 starch/bread, 3 meat, $^1/_2$ fat

Orange-Glazed Pork Tenderloin

1 lb pork tenderloin, cut into 8 pieces

$^3/_4$ c orange juice

3 Tbsp orange marmalade

3 Tbsp brown sugar

2 Tbsp vinegar

1. Heat large skillet coated with cooking spray over medium-high heat. Add pork and cook 3 minutes per side or until thermometer inserted in center reaches 155°F and juices run clear.

2. In a cup, combine juice, marmalade, sugar, and vinegar. Pour over pork. Cover and simmer 20 minutes.

Makes 4 servings

Per serving: 230 cal, 24 g pro, 25 g carb, 4 g fat, 1.5 g sat fat, 75 mg chol, 0 g fiber, 70 mg sodium

Diet Exchanges: 0 milk, $^1/_2$ fruit, 0 vegetable, 1 starch/bread, $3^1/_2$ meat, $^1/_2$ fat

Lemony Pork Chops

$^1/_3$ c all-purpose flour

1 egg

$^1/_4$ c seasoned dry bread crumbs

1 Tbsp crab-boil seasoning, such as Old Bay

4 boneless pork chops, trimmed of all
    visible fat and pounded to $^1/_4$" thickness

1 Tbsp olive oil

Lemon slices

1. Place flour in shallow dish. Beat egg in another shallow dish. Combine bread crumbs and crab-boil seasoning in third dish. Dredge pork in flour,

shaking off any excess. Coat with egg, then with bread-crumb mixture, coating both sides thoroughly.

2. Heat oil in large nonstick skillet over medium heat. Add chops and cook 7 minutes on each side or until thermometer inserted in center of a chop registers 160°F and juices run clear. Serve topped with lemon slices.

Makes 4 servings

Per serving: 270 cal, 28 g pro, 13 g carb, 10 g fat, 2.5 g sat fat, 140 mg chol, 1 g fiber, 320 mg sodium

Diet Exchanges: 0 milk, 0 vegetable, 0 fruit, 1 starch/bread, 4 meat, 1.5 fat

Mexican Pork Tenderloin

3 cloves garlic

$^1/_2$ med onion, chopped

2 chipotle chile peppers canned in adobo sauce, finely chopped

3 Tbsp cider vinegar

2 Tbsp freshly squeezed orange juice

1 Tbsp sugar

2 tsp canola oil

1 tsp chopped fresh oregano

$1^1/_2$ lb pork tenderloin

$^1/_2$ tsp ground cumin

$^1/_2$ tsp salt

$^1/_4$ tsp freshly ground black pepper

1. Caramelize garlic and onion in small dry skillet over medium-high heat, 7 minutes. Transfer to blender. Add chile peppers, vinegar, orange juice, sugar, oil, and oregano and puree. Reserve and chill 3 tablespoons of the marinade. Place pork in shallow dish and cover with remaining marinade. Chill overnight.

2. Preheat grill to medium-high for indirect heat. If using gas grill, heat one side to high, the other to medium. If using charcoal, push coals to one side.

3. Combine cumin, salt, and black pepper in small bowl. Remove tenderloin from marinade (discard marinade), blot dry with paper towel, and rub with spice mixture.

4. Grill pork over high heat 10 minutes. Move to cooler section of grill and brush with reserved marinade. Cover and grill 10 minutes, basting often with marinade, until thermometer inserted in center reaches 155°F and juices run clear.

Makes 4 servings

Per serving: 258 cal, 36 g pro, 7 g carb, 8.5 g fat, 2 g sat fat, 111 mg chol, 0 g fiber, 413 mg sodium

Diet Exchanges: 0 milk, 0.5 vegetable, 0 fruit, 0 starch/bread, 5 meat, 1 fat

Lamb Shanks with Flageolets

2 Tbsp olive oil

4 sm lamb shanks trimmed of all visible fat (about 3 lb total), each cut into 2 or 3 pieces

1 med leek, white part only, halved lengthwise, sliced thinly crosswise, and washed well to remove grit

1 med carrot, sliced diagonally

1 lg clove garlic, minced

1 c canned no salt diced tomatoes

4 sprigs thyme or $^1/_4$ tsp dried

1 bay leaf

4 c low-fat reduced-sodium chicken broth

2 c unsalted canned flageolets or navy beans, rinsed and drained

1. Preheat oven to 350°F.

2. Heat oil in heavy 6-quart, ovenproof Dutch oven over medium-high heat. Add lamb, season with freshly ground black pepper, and brown on all sides, about 15 minutes. Transfer lamb to platter.

3. Add leek, carrot, and garlic to Dutch oven and cook, stirring frequently, for 2 minutes or until vegetables begin to soften. Stir in tomatoes (with juice), thyme, and bay leaf. Add lamb and broth and bring to a simmer.

4. Cover Dutch oven and place on middle rack of oven. Cook $2^1/_2$ to 3 hours or until meat is tender. Stir in beans 15 minutes before end of cooking time. Remove bay leaf before serving.

Makes 6 servings

Per serving: 342 cal, 41 g pro, 19 g carb, 11 g fat, 3 g sat fat, 105 mg chol, 6 g fiber, 573 mg sodium

Diet Exchanges: 0 milk, 1 vegetable, 0 fruit, 0.5 starch/bread, 5.5 meat, 1.5 fat

Grilled Lamb Chops with Mint

$1^1/_2$ c whole-milk plain yogurt

$1^1/_4$ c loosely packed fresh mint leaves

Freshly grated zest of 1 lemon

Freshly squeezed juice of 1 lemon

1 Tbsp garam masala

$^1/_2$ tsp salt

$1^1/_2$ lb frenched lamb rib chops (about 12), $^1/_2$" to $^3/_4$" thick

1. Combine yogurt, mint, lemon zest, lemon juice, and garam masala in food processor or blender. Pulse 2 or 3 times or until blended. Season with salt and freshly ground black pepper to taste.

2. Scoop half of the yogurt mixture into shallow baking dish. Add lamb and flip to coat both sides. Cover and chill

2 hours, turning once. Reserve remaining yogurt mixture.

3. Heat grill to medium-high. Remove chops from marinade. Discard leftover marinade. Place chops over hottest part of grill and cook about 5 minutes, turning once, or until browned and thermometer inserted in center registers 145°F for medium-rare. Arrange lamb on large warm platter, cover, and let rest 5 minutes. Serve with reserved yogurt sauce.

Makes 6 servings

Per serving: 118 cal, 12 g pro, 4 g carb, 6 g fat, 2.5 g sat fat, 37 mg chol, 1 g fiber, 201 mg sodium

Diet Exchanges: 0 milk, 0 vegetable, 0 fruit, 0 starch/bread, 1.5 meat, 0.5 fat

Hoisin-Glazed Leg of Lamb

2 Tbsp hoisin sauce

4 tsp packed chopped cilantro leaves

1 tsp hot sesame oil

1 tsp minced garlic

$1/4$ tsp salt

$1/4$ tsp black pepper

2 lb boneless leg of lamb (ask butcher to remove visible fat)

1. Preheat oven to 400°F.

2. In medium shallow bowl, whisk hoisin sauce, cilantro, oil, garlic, salt, and pepper until combined. Add lamb and turn to coat all sides.

3. Coat baking or roasting pan just larger than roast with olive oil spray. Place roast in pan. Add 2 tablespoons water to bottom of pan. Roast, basting occasionally, 30 to 40 minutes or until thermometer inserted in center registers 145°F for medium-rare/160°F for medium/160°F for well-done. Transfer to serving platter and let stand 10 minutes. Slice.

Makes 8 servings

Per serving: 160 cal, 21 g pro, 2 g carb, 7 g fat, 2.5 g sat fat, 70 mg chol, 0 g fiber, 190 mg sodium

Diet Exchanges: 0 milk, 0 vegetable, 0 fruit, 0 starch/bread, 3 meat, 1 fat

FISH AND SEAFOOD MAIN DISHES

Chile-Lime Snapper

2 Tbsp olive oil

1 bunch fresh basil, coarsely chopped

1 Thai or serrano chile pepper, finely
    chopped (wear plastic gloves when
    handling)

1 lb red snapper fillets

1 lime

1. Heat oil in large skillet over medium heat. Add basil and pepper and cook 1 minute. Remove from pan and set aside.

2. Add fish to pan. Squeeze juice from lime over fish and sprinkle with salt and black pepper to taste.

3. Cover and cook 5 minutes. Turn fish and season with additional black pepper. Return the basil and pepper to the pan. Cover and cook 3 minutes or until fish is opaque.

Makes 4 servings

Per serving: 181 cal, 23 g pro, 1 g carb, 8 g fat, 1.5 g sat fat, 45 mg chol, 0 g fiber, 130 mg sodium

Diet Exchanges: 0 milk, 0 vegetable, 0 fruit, 0 starch/bread, 3 meat, 1^1/$_2$ fat

Mustard Salmon Steaks

4 salmon steaks (5 oz each)

2 Tbsp maple syrup

1 Tbsp mustard

1 Tbsp minced onion

^{1}/$_2$ tsp dried dill

1 c cooked whole wheat couscous

1. Preheat oven to 400°F.

2. Place steaks in nonstick baking dish. Combine syrup, mustard, and onion, and drizzle or brush over steaks. Sprinkle dill over glaze.

3. Bake, uncovered, 20 minutes or until fish is just opaque. Serve over couscous.

Makes 4 servings

Per serving: 282 cal, 30 g pro, 18 g carb, 9.4 g fat, 1.4 g sat fat, 78 mg chol, 2 g fiber, 106 mg sodium

Diet Exchanges: 0 milk, 0 vegetable, 0 fruit, 2.5 starch/bread, 4 meat, 0 fat

Seared Wild Salmon with Mango Salsa

Photo on page 353

Salsa

1 ripe mango, peeled and cut into small
    cubes (about $1^1/_2$ c)

$^1/_2$ c chopped red bell pepper

$^1/_2$ c chopped red onion

3 Tbsp freshly squeezed lime juice

2 Tbsp chopped fresh mint

1 Tbsp finely chopped jalapeño chile pepper

Salmon

Juice of 1 lemon (about $^1/_4$ c)

$^1/_2$ tsp paprika

2 wild salmon fillets (1 lb each, about
    1" thick)

1 Tbsp olive oil

1. To prepare salsa: Toss together mango, bell pepper, onion, lime juice, mint, and jalapeño chile pepper in small bowl. Season with salt and freshly ground black pepper to taste. Cover and chill at least 1 hour to blend flavors.

2. To prepare salmon: Combine lemon juice and paprika in large shallow baking dish. Season with salt and freshly ground black pepper. Place salmon in dish and flip to cover both sides. Marinate, covered, up to 1 hour in refrigerator.

3. Remove fillets from marinade. Discard marinade. Heat oil in large nonstick skillet over medium-high heat. Sear fillets 15 minutes, turning once, or until opaque. Serve with salsa.

Makes 6 servings

Per serving: 272 cal, 31 g pro, 10 g carb, 12 g fat, 2 g sat fat, 83 mg chol, 1 g fiber, 69 mg sodium

Diet Exchanges: 0 milk, 0.5 vegetable, 0.5 fruit, 0 starch/bread, 4 meat, 0.5 fat

Savory Salmon Brunch Skillet

$^2/_3$ c fat-free sour cream

1 tsp freshly squeezed lemon juice

$2^1/_2$ Tbsp chopped fresh dill

1 Tbsp olive oil

1 pkg (28 oz) frozen diced potatoes with onions and peppers (i.e., "O'Brien" potatoes)

2 c flaked Seared Wild Salmon (about $^1/_2$ lb) (see page 337)

$^1/_3$ c chopped scallions

1 tsp Dijon mustard

1. Blend sour cream, lemon juice, and $1^1/_2$ tablespoons of the dill in small bowl. Season with salt and freshly ground black pepper. Set aside.

2. Coat large nonstick skillet with cooking spray. Add oil and heat over medium heat. Spread potatoes evenly over bottom of pan, cover, and cook, stirring occasionally, 10 minutes or until heated through. Remove cover, increase heat to medium-high, and press potatoes with large spatula. Cook 5 minutes or until potatoes brown and begin to crisp, turning occasionally.

3. Combine salmon, scallions, mustard, and the remaining 1 tablespoon dill in medium bowl while potatoes cook. Season with salt and freshly ground black pepper. Add salmon mixture to pan, combining with potatoes by turning sections with spatula (try not to break up potatoes). Cook until heated through, about 2 minutes. Serve with reserved dill cream.

Makes 4 servings

Per serving: 293 cal, 13 g pro, 46 g carb, 7 g fat, 1.5 g sat fat, 23 mg chol, 5 g fiber, 149 mg sodium

Diet Exchanges: 0 milk, 0 vegetable, 0 fruit, 2 starch/bread, 1 meat, 1 fat

Wasabi Salmon Sandwiches

$^1/_4$ c fat-free mayonnaise

$^1/_4$–$^1/_2$ tsp wasabi paste (sold in ethnic-food section of most supermarkets)

2 c flaked Seared Wild Salmon (about $^1/_2$ lb) (see page 337)

8 thin slices ($^1/_2$ oz each) whole wheat bread, toasted

4 thin slices red onion

4 thin red bell pepper rings

4 Tbsp sliced pickled ginger

1 c arugula

1. Combine mayonnaise and wasabi paste in small bowl until smooth. Start with $1/4$ teaspoon of the paste and add more to suit your taste. Gently fold in salmon.

2. Place 4 slices of the bread on flat surface and top each with $1/2$ cup of the salmon mixture, 1 onion slice (separated and evenly spread over salmon), 1 pepper ring, 1 tablespoon of the ginger, and $1/4$ cup of the arugula. Top with remaining 4 slices of bread.

Makes 4 servings

Per serving: 185 cal, 11 g pro, 23 g carb, 4.5 g fat, 0.5 g sat fat, 21 mg chol, 4 g fiber, 361 mg sodium

Diet Exchanges: 0 milk, 0.5 vegetable, 0 fruit, 1 starch/bread, 1 meat, 0.5 fat

Lemony Stuffed Sole

1 lb sole or flounder fillets

$1/4$ tsp salt

$1/8$ tsp freshly ground black pepper

1 c Summer Squash Sauté (see page 299)

1 tsp extra-virgin olive oil

$1/4$ c dry white wine, or 2 Tbsp freshly squeezed lemon juice mixed with 2 Tbsp vegetable broth

1 Tbsp butter

2 tsp freshly squeezed lemon juice

$1/2$ tsp freshly grated lemon zest

1 tsp finely chopped fresh parsley

1. Season both sides of fish with salt and pepper. Place 1 fillet on flat surface and spread 2 tablespoons of the squash evenly over top, leaving a $1/2$" margin on both ends. Starting with one end, roll fillet into a cylinder and secure with wooden pick. Repeat with remaining sole and squash.

2. Heat oil in 12" nonstick skillet over medium heat and add sole, seam side up. Cook 2 minutes and add wine or lemon juice and broth. Reduce heat to medium-low, cover, and cook 5 minutes longer or until fish is opaque.

3. Transfer sole to a plate and tent loosely with foil. Add butter, lemon juice, and lemon zest to skillet. Remove from heat, swirl until butter melts, and spoon over sole. Sprinkle with parsley. Remove pick before serving.

Makes 4 servings

Per serving: 171 cal, 20 g pro, 4 g carb, 7 g fat, 2.5 g sat fat, 61 mg chol, 1 g fiber, 323 mg sodium

Diet Exchanges: 0 milk, 0.5 vegetable, 0 fruit, 0 starch/bread, 3 meat, 1 fat

Thai Sweet-Hot Shrimp

3 cloves garlic, minced

1 serrano chile pepper, minced (wear plastic
   gloves when handling)

1½ Tbsp reduced-sodium fish sauce

1½ Tbsp sugar

1 Tbsp freshly squeezed orange juice

1 Tbsp rice wine vinegar

½ tsp chile paste (available in ethnic-food
   section of most supermarkets)

1½ lb lg shrimp, shelled, deveined, and
   patted dry

1. Combine garlic, pepper, fish sauce, sugar, orange juice, vinegar, and chile paste in small saucepan and bring to a boil. Reduce heat to medium and simmer 3 minutes or until mixture thickens slightly. Let cool.

2. Place shrimp in large bowl. Add 3 tablespoons of marinade, tossing well to coat shrimp and rubbing into flesh. Chill 30 minutes. Reserve remaining marinade.

3. Coat grill rack with cooking spray and preheat grill to medium-high.

4. Skewer shrimp and grill 3 to 4 minutes or until opaque, turning once and brushing with reserved marinade.

Makes 6 servings

Per serving: 139 cal, 23 g pro, 5 g carb, 2 g fat, 0.5 g sat fat, 172 mg chol, 0 g fiber, 394 mg sodium

Diet Exchanges: 0 milk, 0 vegetable, 0 fruit, 0 starch/bread, 3 meat, 0 fat

Chai Scallops with Bok Choy

Photo on page 354

2 chai tea bags (we used Yogi Tea)

2–4 heads baby bok choy (12 oz), quartered
    lengthwise or halved if sm

1 Tbsp finely chopped fresh ginger

1 lb sea scallops, each halved across grain
    to form 2 disks

$^1/_4$ tsp salt

2 tsp canola oil

$^1/_3$ c light coconut milk

1 lime, cut into 4 wedges

1. Steep tea bags 3 minutes in $^1/_3$ cup boiling water. Discard tea bags. Set aside tea.

2. Sprinkle bok choy with ginger. Steam over rapidly boiling water in steamer with lid about 8 minutes or until bright green and easily pierced with tip of knife.

3. Pat scallops dry and sprinkle with salt. Warm oil in large skillet over medium-high heat. Add scallops in a single layer. (Work in batches if necessary.) Cook 2 minutes on each side or until opaque, and set aside.

4. Add reserved tea and coconut milk to skillet. Cook, swirling pan and allowing chai sauce to thicken. Divide sauce among 4 shallow bowls. Top with bok choy and reserved scallops. Serve with lime wedges to squeeze over scallops.

Makes 4 servings

Per serving: 150 cal, 21 g pro, 7 g carb, 4.5 g fat, 1.5 g sat fat, 37 mg chol, 1 g fiber, 389 mg sodium

Diet Exchanges: 0 milk, 0.5 vegetable, 0 fruit, 0 starch/bread, 3 meat, 0.5 fat

DESSERTS

Apple Crisp

Photo on page 355

Topping

$^1/_2$ c all-purpose flour

3 Tbsp brown sugar

$1^1/_2$ tsp granulated sugar

3 Tbsp butter, at room temperature

Filling

2 lb apples (or other fruit such as peaches), peeled, cored, and sliced (about 6 c + additional slices for garnish)

$^1/_2$ tsp freshly squeezed lemon juice

$^1/_4$ tsp lemon zest

$1^1/_2$ Tbsp granulated sugar (optional)

1. Preheat oven to 375°F.

2. To prepare topping: In medium bowl, combine flour and sugars. Cut butter into small pieces and add. Mix in butter by rubbing it in flour mixture lightly and quickly between fingertips until evenly combined and mixture looks crumbly.

3. To prepare filling: In large bowl, combine apples with lemon juice, lemon zest, and sugar, if using. Transfer to 1-quart glass or ceramic baking dish, spreading to cover bottom. Sprinkle topping evenly over apples. Bake on middle rack about 40 minutes or until topping is brown and apples are soft and bubbly. Cool 10 minutes before serving. Garnish with apple slices, if desired.

Makes 6 servings

Per serving: 162 cal, 1 g pro, 27 g carb, 6 g fat, 3.6 g sat fat, 15 mg chol, 2 g fiber, 42 mg sodium

Diet Exchanges: 0 milk, 0 vegetable, 1 fruit, 1 starch/bread, 0 meat, 1 fat

Sautéed Bananas with Praline Sauce

$^1/_4$ c + $1^1/_2$ Tbsp maple syrup

3 Tbsp fat-free milk

3 Tbsp chopped pecans

4 lg bananas, halved lengthwise and sliced

1. Bring maple syrup, milk, and pecans to a boil in small saucepan over medium-high heat. Reduce heat to medium-low and simmer 10 minutes or until mixture thickens and reduces to about $^1/_3$ cup.

2. Heat large nonstick skillet coated with cooking spray over medium-high heat. Add bananas and cook, stirring frequently, 2 minutes.

3. Place bananas in serving dish and top with sauce.

Makes 8 servings

Per serving: 120 cal, 1 g pro, 25 g carb, 2.2 g fat, 0 g sat fat, 0 mg chol, 2 g fiber, 4 mg sodium

Diet Exchanges: 0 milk, 0 vegetable, 1 fruit, 0.5 starch/bread, 0 meat, 0.5 fat

Yogurt and Fruit Delight

1 med red-skinned apple, cut into bite-size chunks

1 can (8 oz) juice-packed pineapple chunks or tidbits

$^1/_4$ c mini marshmallows

6 oz fat-free vanilla yogurt

1 Tbsp chopped nuts, such as pecans or almonds

1. In large bowl, combine apple, pineapple (with juice), and marshmallows. Stir well. Cover and chill at least 6 hours to blend flavors.

2. Drain excess juice. Top with yogurt and sprinkle with nuts.

Makes 3 servings

Per serving: 134 cal, 4 g pro, 27 g carb, 2 g fat, 0 g sat fat, 1 mg chol, 3 g fiber, 43 mg sodium

Diet Exchanges: 0 milk, 0 vegetable, 1 fruit, 1 starch/bread, 0 meat, 0.5 fat

No-Bake Cherry Cheese Pie

6 oz reduced-fat cream cheese

$^3/_4$ c fat-free sour cream

$^1/_4$ c fat-free milk

1 pkg (1 oz) instant sugar-free vanilla pudding mix

1 prepared reduced-fat graham cracker pie crust (9")

1 can (20 oz) light cherry pie filling

1. In blender, combine cream cheese, sour cream, and milk. Process to mix thoroughly. Place in large bowl. Stir in pudding mix. Pour mixture into piecrust and smooth the top. Top with pie filling.

2. Cover and refrigerate at least 2 hours before serving.

Makes 8 servings

Per serving: 204 cal, 6 g pro, 51 g carb, 9 g fat, 3 g sat fat, 5 mg chol, 0 g fiber, 500 mg sodium

Diet Exchanges: 0.5 milk, 0 vegetable, 1 fruit, 2 starch/bread, 0 meat, 1.5 fat

Fruit Sundae

8 oz fat-free frozen whipped topping,
    thawed

1 sheets reduced-fat cinnamon graham
    crackers, coarsely crumbled

1 c strawberries, sliced

1 Tbsp chocolate syrup

1. Divide one-third of topping among 4 dessert bowls. Sprinkle one-third of the graham crackers, one-third of the strawberries, and 1 teaspoon of the syrup evenly among bowls. Repeat layering 2 more times to use remaining ingredients.

2. Cover and freeze 2 hours or until hardened. Serve frozen or allow to thaw slightly.

Makes 4 servings

Per serving: 135 cal, 1 g pro, 28 g carb, 0.5 g fat, 0 g sat fat, 0 mg chol, 1 g fiber, 56 mg sodium

Diet Exchanges: 0 milk, 0 vegetable, 0.5 fruit, 1 starch/bread, 0 meat, 0 fat

Cardamom Shortcakes with Mangoes

2 ripe mangoes, peeled and cut into
    $1/2$" cubes

2 Tbsp honey

1.5 tsp freshly grated lime zest

1.5 tsp freshly squeezed lime juice

$1/3$ c heavy cream

6 Cardamom Biscuits (see page 287)

6 fresh mint leaves

1. Place mangoes, honey, lime zest, and lime juice in top half of double boiler over medium-high heat. (You can simulate a double boiler by fitting a bowl into a larger saucepot filled with water.) Simmer, stirring occasionally, about 8 minutes or until mango cubes are softened. Set aside to cool.

2. Whisk cream in small bowl until soft peaks form. To assemble shortcakes, split biscuits with fork. Spoon $1/4$ cup of the mangoes over bottom half of biscuit. Top with other half, a dollop of whipped cream, another $1/4$ cup of the mangoes, and a mint leaf. Repeat with remaining ingredients.

Makes 6 servings

Per serving: 180 cal, 3 g pro, 30 g carb, 6.5 g fat, 2 g sat fat, 10 mg chol, 3 g fiber, 110 mg sodium

Diet Exchanges: 0 milk, 0 vegetable, 0.5 fruit, 1 starch/bread, 0 meat, 1 fat

Strawberry Pie

1 can (20 oz) strawberry pie filling

1 pt fresh or thawed frozen strawberries, hulled and sliced, with some reserved for garnish

1 prepared reduced fat graham cracker piecrust (9")

8 oz frozen whipped topping, thawed

1. Alternately layer pie filling and strawberries in piecrust. Top with whipped topping. Garnish with strawberry slices.

2. Cover and refrigerate at least 1 hour before serving.

Makes 12 servings

Per serving: 171 cal, 2 g pro, 27 g carb, 5.6 g fat, 3.5 g sat fat, 0 mg chol, 1 g fiber, 57 mg sodium

Diet Exchanges: 0 milk, 0 vegetable, 0.5 fruit, 1.5 starch/bread, 0 meat, 0.5 fat

Piña Colada Cake

1 pkg ($14\frac{1}{2}$ oz) angel food cake mix

1 can (8 oz) juice-packed crushed pineapple

8 oz fat-free frozen whipped topping, thawed

$\frac{1}{2}$ c toasted coconut (2 oz)

1. Preheat oven to 350°F. Coat 13" × 9" baking dish with cooking spray.

2. In large bowl, combine cake mix and pineapple. Pour into baking dish.

3. Bake 20 minutes or until wooden pick inserted in center comes out almost clean. Cool completely on a rack.

4. Evenly spread topping over cake. Sprinkle with coconut. Cover and refrigerate until ready to serve.

Makes 16 servings

Per serving: 150 cal, 3 g pro, 30 g carb, 2 g fat, 1.5 g sat fat, 0 mg chol, 0 g fiber, 200 mg sodium

Diet Exchanges: 0 milk, 0 vegetable, 0 fruit, 2 starch/bread, 0 meat, 0.5 fat

Pumpkin-Maple Cheesecake

Photo on page 356

3 pkg (8 oz) fat-free cream cheese, at room
temperature

$^2/_3$ c packed brown sugar

3 lg eggs

1 can (15 oz) pumpkin puree

$^1/_2$ c low-fat maple or vanilla yogurt

2 Tbsp all-purpose flour

$1^1/_2$ tsp ground cinnamon

1 tsp ground ginger

1 tsp imitation maple or rum flavoring

1 tsp pure vanilla extract

$^1/_4$ c minced crystallized ginger (optional)

1. Preheat oven to 350°F. Assemble 9" springform pan and coat with cooking spray.

2. Using electric mixer, beat cream cheese and sugar until smooth. Beat in eggs one at a time. Blend in pumpkin, yogurt, flour, cinnamon, ginger, flavoring, and vanilla extract.

3. Pour filling into pan. Bake until outer rim is puffy and center is slightly wobbly, about 1 hour 10 minutes. Remove from oven and run knife around side to loosen. Let stand at room temperature 30 minutes. Refrigerate warm cake, uncovered, until cold. Then cover with foil and refrigerate at least 4 hours (or up to 3 days). Remove 1 hour before serving.

4. When ready to serve, carefully remove side of pan. Cut into wedges with wet knife wiped clean between cuts. Garnish with crystallized ginger, if desired.

Makes 12 servings

Per serving: 150 cal, 11 g pro, 22 g carb, 1.5 g fat, 0.5 g sat fat, 65 mg chol, 1 g fiber, 310 mg sodium

Diet Exchanges: 0 milk, 0 vegetable, 0 fruit, 1.5 starch/bread, 1.5 meat, 0 fat

Chocolate–Peanut Butter Pie

Photo on page 357

$1^3/_4$ c fat-free milk

$^1/_2$ c reduced-fat peanut butter (not fat-free because it won't set up)

1 pkg (1.3 oz) instant sugar-free chocolate pudding mix

8 oz light frozen whipped topping, thawed

1 prepared reduced-fat graham cracker or chocolate cookie piecrust (9")

Chocolate shavings (optional)

1. In large microwaveable bowl, combine milk and peanut butter. Cover

with plastic wrap and microwave on medium 3 minutes or until peanut butter is melted. Stir until smooth. Add pudding mix and stir until thickened. Gently fold in topping. Spoon mixture into piecrust and smooth the top. Cover and refrigerate overnight.

2. Top each serving with chocolate shavings, if using. Serve chilled.

Makes 8 servings

Per serving: 240 cal, 7 g pro, 30 g carb, 11 g fat, 3 g sat fat, 0 mg chol, 1 g fiber, 440 mg sodium

Diet Exchanges: 0.5 milk, 0 vegetable, 0 fruit, 0.5 bread, 0.5 meat, 1.5 fat

Chocolate Ice Milk Sundaes

Ice milk

$^3/_4$ c superfine sugar

$^1/_3$ c unsweetened cocoa powder

2 c cold 1% milk

$^1/_2$ tsp pure vanilla extract

Sauce

$^1/_3$ c granulated sugar substitute

3 Tbsp unsweetened cocoa powder

$^1/_3$ c strong brewed coffee or espresso

1 tsp pure vanilla extract

1. To prepare ice milk: In large bowl, whisk together sugar and cocoa. Slowly whisk in milk and vanilla extract until dry ingredients are dissolved and no lumps remain.

2. Pour into 8" × 8" baking pan. Freeze about $1^1/_2$ hours or until nearly frozen.

3. Score the surface with a sharp knife and cut into chunks. Transfer to food processor or blender and process until smooth and creamy.

4. Pour into a resealable container. Freeze 2 to 3 hours or until very firm.

5. To prepare sauce: In small saucepan, combine sugar substitute and cocoa. Stir in coffee or espresso. Bring to a boil over medium heat, stirring. Reduce heat to low and cook 8 minutes or until slightly thickened. Let cool slightly and stir in vanilla extract. Serve over scoops of ice milk.

Makes 6 servings

Per serving: 146 cal, 4 g pro, 32 g carb, 2 g fat, 1 g sat fat, 4 mg chol, 2 g fiber, 38 mg sodium

Diet Exchanges: 0.5 milk, 0 vegetable, 0 fruit, 2 starch/bread, 0 meat, 0 fat

Enlightened Brownies

$1/2$ c cake flour

$1/2$ c unsweetened cocoa powder

$1/4$ tsp baking powder

$1/4$ tsp salt

1 lg egg

2 lg egg whites

$3/4$ c sugar

$1/2$ c vegetable oil

$1^1/_2$ tsp pure vanilla extract

2 Tbsp chopped pistachios or walnuts

1. Preheat oven to 350°F. Coat 8" × 8" baking pan with cooking spray.

2. In medium bowl, sift together flour, cocoa, baking powder, and salt. In large bowl, whisk egg and egg whites until frothy. Whisk in sugar, oil, and vanilla extract until smooth.

3. Gradually fold in flour mixture until just blended. Pour into prepared pan. Sprinkle with pistachios.

4. Bake 20 to 25 minutes or until wooden pick inserted in center comes out with moist crumbs. Cool in pan on rack and then cut into 12 squares.

Makes 12 brownies

Per brownie: 170 cal, 2 g pro, 18 g carb, 11 g fat, 1.5 g sat fat, 18 mg chol, 1g fiber, 74 mg sodium

Diet Exchanges: 0 milk, 0 vegetable, 0 fruit, 1.5 starch/bread, 0 meat, 2 fat

Chocolate-Nut Torte with Raspberry Glaze

1 c natural (skin on) almonds or walnuts

1 c sugar, divided

2 lg eggs, at room temperature

2 lg egg whites, at room temperature

1 tsp pure vanilla extract

$3/4$ c light olive oil

$3/4$ c all-purpose flour

$1/2$ c unsweetened cocoa powder

1 tsp baking powder

$1/8$ tsp salt

$1/4$ c seedless raspberry fruit spread

1. Preheat oven to 350°F. Coat 10" springform pan with cooking spray. Sprinkle with flour, shake to coat, and tap out excess.

2. In food processor, finely chop almonds with 2 tablespoons of the sugar. Set aside.

3. In large bowl, with electric mixer at medium-high speed, beat eggs, egg whites, and vanilla extract until foamy.

Gradually beat in remaining sugar, 1 tablespoon at a time, until mixture is thick and pale in color, about 5 minutes. Turn mixer to lowest speed and add oil in slow, steady stream.

4. In large bowl, sift together flour, cocoa, baking powder, and salt. Fold in almond mixture. Gradually fold in egg mixture. Pour into prepared pan.

5. Bake 30 to 35 minutes or until edges begin to pull away from pan sides and center is firm to the touch. Cool in pan on rack.

6. In small saucepan over low heat, melt fruit spread until smooth. Spread over cake and let stand 30 minutes or until spread is set. Remove torte from pan before serving.

Makes 12 servings

Per serving: 320 cal, 6g pro, 30 g carb, 22 g fat, 3 g sat fat, 35 mg chol, 3 g fiber, 85 mg sodium

Diet Exchanges: 0 milk, 0 vegetable, 0 fruit, 2 starch/bread, 1 meat, 4 fat

Chocolate-Almond Pudding with Amaretti

$1/3$ c sugar substitute

$1/3$ c unsweetened cocoa powder

2 Tbsp + 2 tsp cornstarch

2 c 1% milk

1 tsp pure vanilla extract

$1/4$ tsp almond extract

8 almond-flavored cookies, crushed (about $1/3$ c)

1. In medium saucepan, sift together sugar substitute, cocoa, and cornstarch. Gradually stir in milk until cornstarch dissolves. Bring to a boil over medium-low heat, stirring gently. Cook, stirring, 6 minutes or until thickened and smooth. Remove from heat. Stir in vanilla and almond extracts.

2. Spoon half of pudding mixture into four 4-ounce ramekins, wineglasses, or parfait glasses. Sprinkle with half of the cookies. Top with remaining pudding and cookies and serve.

Makes 4 servings

Per serving: 203 cal, 7 g pro, 27 g carb, 8 g fat, 2.5 g sat fat, 15 mg chol, 3 g fiber, 103 mg sodium

Diet Exchanges: 0.5 milk, 0 vegetable, 0 fruit, 1.5 starch/bread, 0 meat, 1.5 fat

Chocolate Bliss Bites

Photo on page 358

> $^{1}/_{2}$ c unsweetened cocoa powder
>
> Pinch of salt
>
> $^{1}/_{2}$ c sugar, divided
>
> 3 lg egg whites
>
> $^{1}/_{8}$ tsp cream of tartar
>
> 1 tsp pure vanilla extract
>
> 1 Tbsp confectioners' sugar

1. Preheat oven to 300°F. Line 2 baking sheets with foil.

2. In small bowl, sift together cocoa, salt, and $^{1}/_{4}$ cup of the sugar.

3. In large bowl, with electric mixer at medium-low speed, beat egg whites and cream of tartar until soft peaks form. Beat in remaining $^{1}/_{4}$ cup sugar, $^{1}/_{2}$ tablespoon at a time, until meringue is glossy and stiff peaks form. Fold in cocoa mixture and vanilla extract.

4. Drop by rounded teaspoonfuls about 1" apart onto prepared baking sheets. Bake 25 minutes for soft, chewy cookies or 40 minutes for crisp ones. Dust cooled cookies with confectioners' sugar.

Makes 24 cookies

Per cookie: 25 cal, 1 g pro, 6 g carb, 0 g fat, 0 g sat fat, 0 mg chol, 0.5 g fiber, 13mg sodium

Diet Exchanges: 0 milk, 0 vegetable, 0 fruit, 0.5 starch/bread, 0 meat, 0 fat

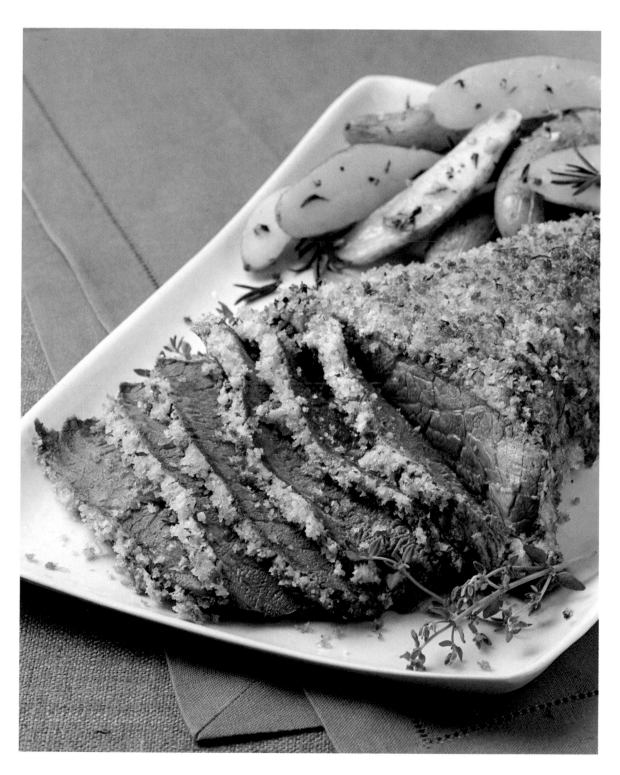

Mustard-Crusted London Broil
Recipe on page 326

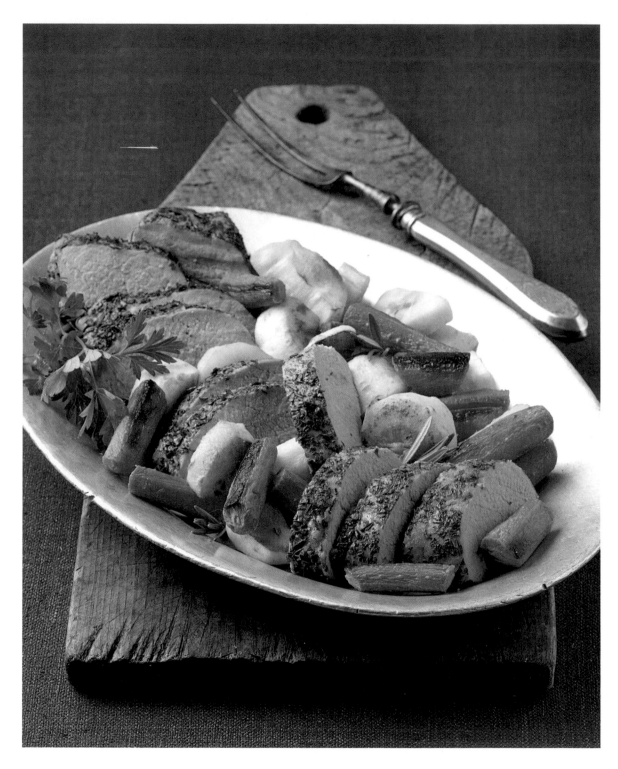

Herbed Pork Roast
Recipe on page 330

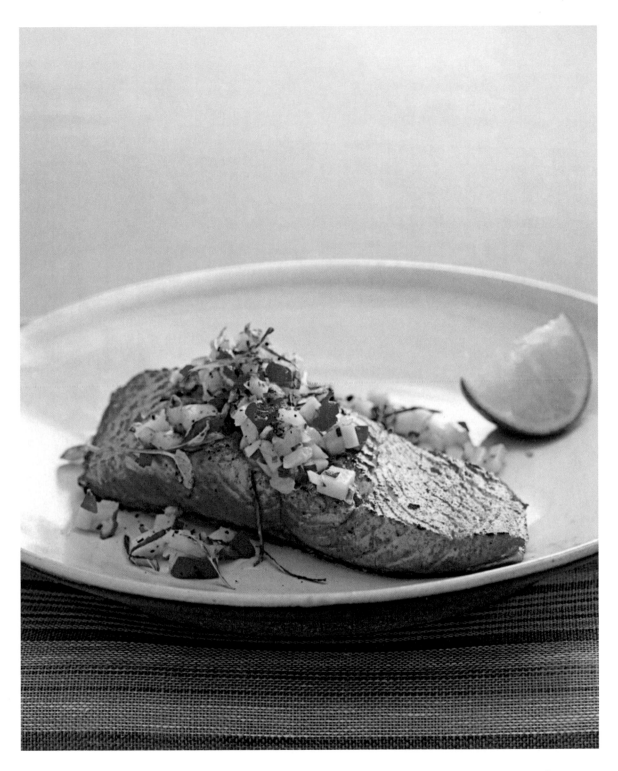

Seared Wild Salmon with Mango Salsa

Recipe on page 337

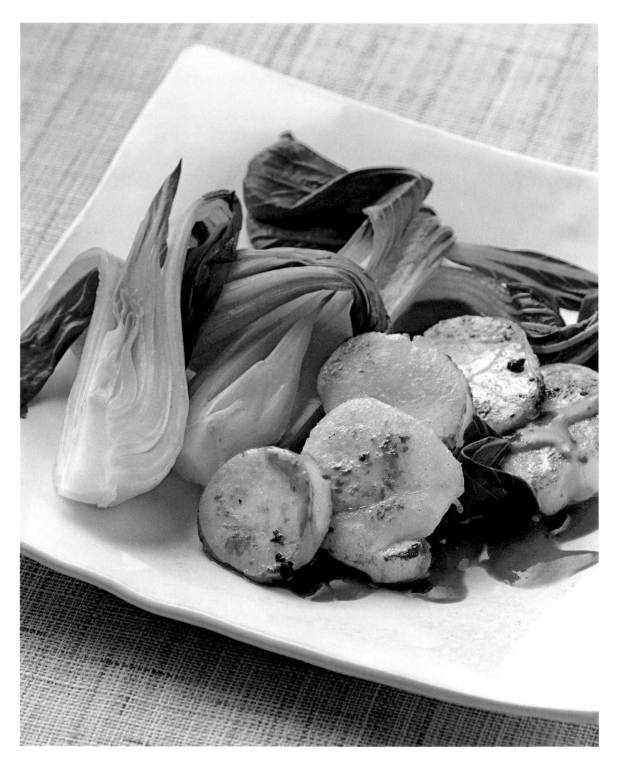

Chai Scallops with Bok Choy
Recipe on page 341

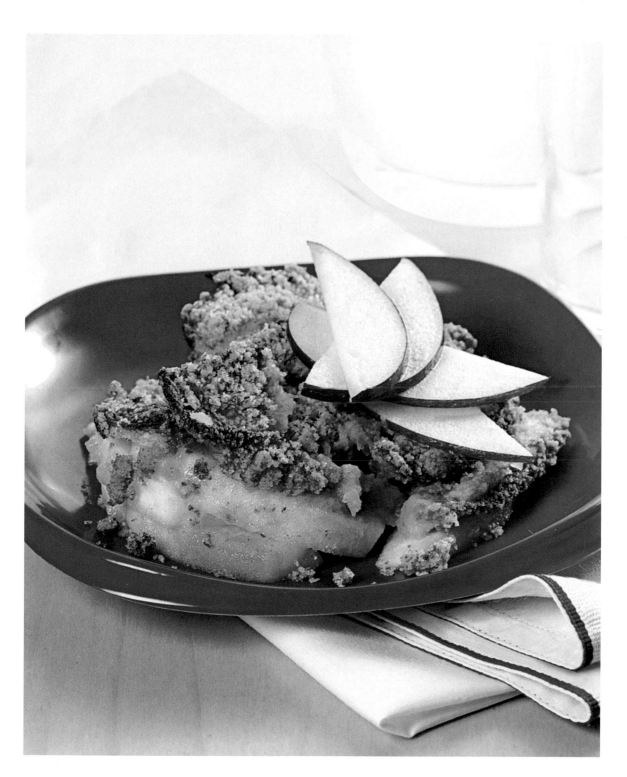

Apple Crisp
Recipe on page 342

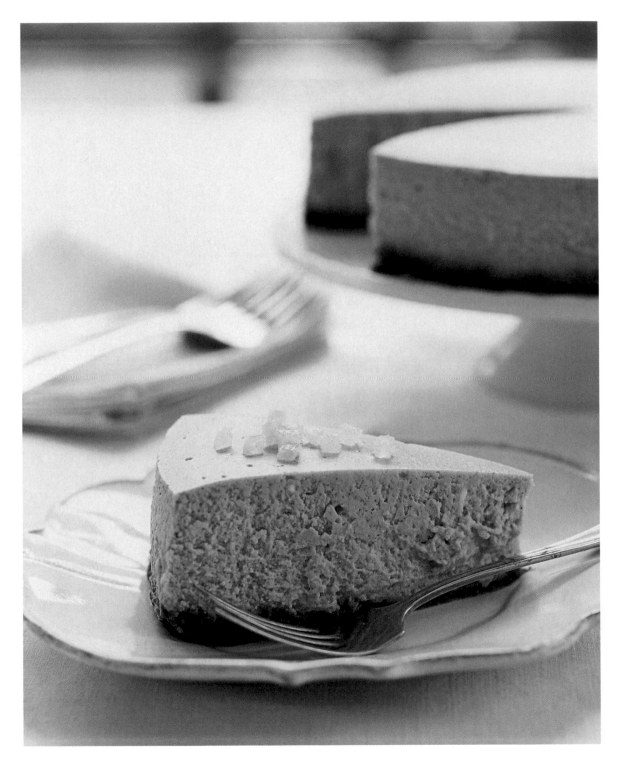

Pumpkin-Maple Cheesecake
Recipe on page 346

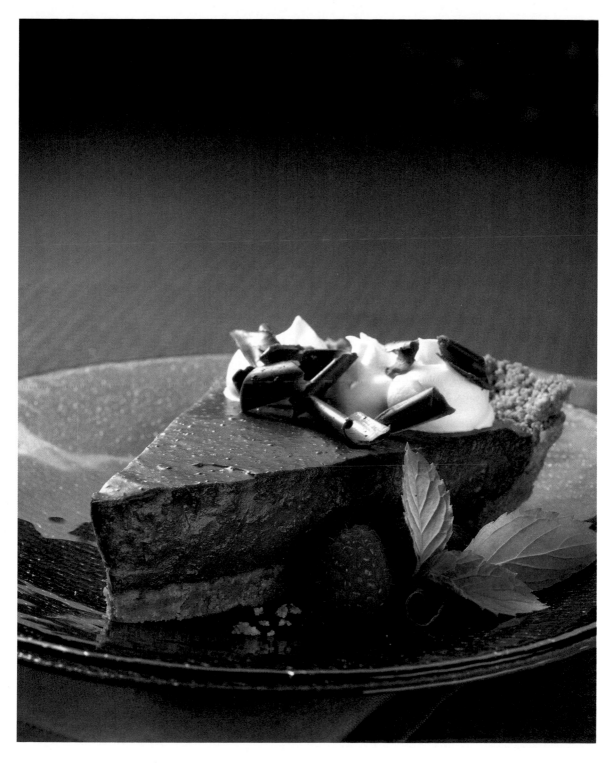

Chocolate Peanut Butter Pie
Recipe on page 346

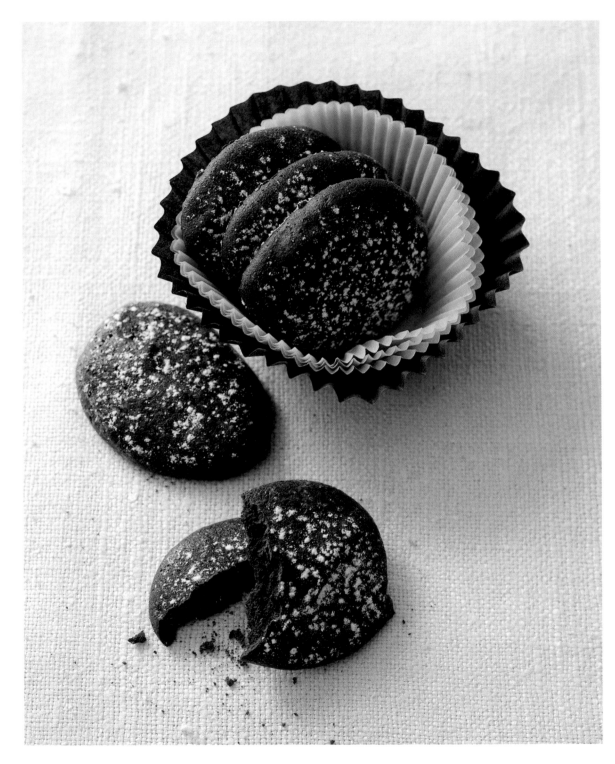

Chocolate Bliss Bites
Recipe on page 350

Photo Credits

Pages 116–123 and 175–180 : © David Martinez

Pages 138–139, 142–145, 168–171, 183–188, and 190–193: © Hilmar

Pages 279, 353, and 358: © Yunhee Kim

Pages 280, 283, and 355: © Brian Hagiwara

Page 281: © Ngo Minh Ngoc

Pages 284, 351, 352, and 354: © Elizabeth Watt

Page 285: © Mark Ferry

Pages 286 and 356: © Alexandra Rowley

Page 357: © Mitch Mandel/Rodale Images

Index

Boldface page references indicate photographs. <u>Underscored</u> references indicate boxed text and charts.

A

Abdominal exercises, 165
Abdominal fat
  diet in reducing, 153–54
  exercise in reducing, 153–54
  heart disease and, <u>250–51</u>
  risk factor of, 26–27
  soda and, 75, 77–78
Acetyl L-carnitine (ALC), 264–65
Acomplia (rimonabant), 27–28
Adiponectin, 26–27
Adult-onset diabetes. *See* Type 2 diabetes
Aerobie AeroPress, 89, 95
Agatston score, 236
Agave nectar, 70
Ala54Thr gene, 47
ALC, 264–65
Alcohol. *See also* Wine
  beer, <u>61</u>
  breast cancer and, 90
  cancer risk and, 90, <u>241</u>, 261
  dependence, 90
  diabetes and, <u>61</u>
  as diet derailment, 130–31
  serving glasses for, 150
Alcoholism, 90
Alertness, <u>205</u>
Alliinase, 92
Alternative medicine, 41
Amino acids, 85, 140
Anger management, 219–22, <u>221</u>
Antidepressants, 253–56, <u>254</u>
Antioxidants, 63, 69, 88, 94, 261
Artificial sweeteners, <u>76</u>
Atkins diet, 21

Attitude, adjusting, 214–18
Autoimmune disease, 33. *See also* Type 1
  diabetes

B

Balding, 48–49
Beef
  grilling, 93
  Hearty Beef-Vegetable Soup, 295
  Korean Barbecued Beef, 327
  Moroccan Meatballs in Tomato Sauce, 329
  Mustard-Crusted London Broil, 326–27,
    351
  Spiced Kofta Sliders, 328
  Vietnamese Beef Salad, **281**, 288
Beer, <u>61</u>
Beta-carotene, 91, 93
Beta cells, 33–34, <u>36</u>
Beverages. *See also* Coffee; Soda
  beer, <u>61</u>
  Bring-on-the-Morning Smoothie, 275
  Frothy Hot Chocolate, 275, **279**
  fruit juices, 75, 79
  milkshakes, <u>81</u>
  sports drinks, 73, 79
  sugar-free, <u>76</u>
  water, 9, <u>76</u>, <u>81</u>
Bingeing, avoiding, <u>205</u>
Blood clotting, 49
Blood platelets, 64
Blood pressure, 26, 88, 197, 242, <u>251</u>
Blood sugar level. *See also* Glucose
  balancing, 7–8
  carbohydrates and, 20
  chromium and, 65